Life Inside the "Thin" Cage

A Personal Look

into the Hidden World

of the Chronic Dieter

Constance Rhodes

Foreword by Karyn H. Williams, Ph.D.

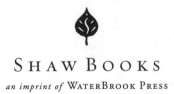

SHAW BOOKS

an imprint of WATERBROOK PRESS

Life Inside the "Thin" Cage
A SHAW BOOK
PUBLISHED BY WATERBROOK PRESS
2375 Telstar Drive, Suite 160
Colorado Springs, Colorado 80920
A division of Random House, Inc.

All Scripture quotations, unless otherwise indicated, are taken from *The Holy Bible, New Century Version,* copyright © 1987, 1988, 1991 by Word Publishing, Nashville, TN 37214. Used by permission.

This book is not intended to replace the medical advice of a trained medical professional. Readers are advised to consult a physician or other qualified health-care professional regarding treatment of their medical problems. The author and publisher specifically disclaim liability, loss, or risk, personal or otherwise, that may be incurred as a consequence, directly or indirectly, in the use or application of any of the contents of this book.

Details and names in some stories and illustrations have been changed to protect the identities of the persons involved. Some illustrations are a combination of individual stories.

ISBN 0-87788-038-7

SHAW BOOKS and its aspen leaf logo are trademarks of WaterBrook Press, a division of Random House, Inc.

Library of Congress Cataloging-in-Publication Data
Rhodes, Constance.
  Life inside the "thin" cage : a personal look into the hidden world of the chronic dieter / Constance
Rhodes.—1st ed.
    p. cm.
  ISBN 0-87788-038-7
  1. Eating disorders—Popular works. 2. Weight loss—Psychological aspects. 3. Body image in women.
I. Title.
RC552.E18 R53 2003
613.2'5'019—dc21

                                                                              2002153757

Printed in the United States of America
2003—First Edition

10 9 8 7 6 5 4 3 2 1

*This book is dedicated to the millions of women
who have sacrificed their time, energy, health, and happiness
to appease the "goddess of thin."
May you find freedom from your cages.*

Contents

Acknowledgments

The more help a person has in his garden, the less it belongs to him.

—William H. Davies

For a story that spans thirty years, it is impossible to thank all who have played a role. But it is with deepest gratitude that I wish to honor publicly those without whom this book and FINDING *balance* would not exist.

To AJ—God truly sent me an angel in you. Thank you for loving me through the darkest days and for being such an integral part of all that is good in my life. I live each day humbly aware of your willingness to live unselfishly in order that someone else (usually me) will have what their heart desires. You are a wonderful husband, father, and friend, and a most precious gift to me.

To Christian—Your smile and innocence are constant reminders of what is truly important in this life.

To Mom—Your beauty is matched only by the strength of your spirit. Thank you for allowing me to open a window into your private world and for helping guide me through the writing of this book.

To Dad—You have been a constant source of wisdom to me and a visionary from whom I've learned that, with focus and hard work, anything is possible.

To the early encouragers: Brenda Boswell, Lisa Harper, Jackie Russell, Norman Miller, David Huffman, Melissa Hambrick, Becky Sowers, Jen Blaney, Janet Bozeman, Jackie Marushka, DeDe Tarrant—Your support boosted my confidence at a time when I needed it most.

To Kevin Kookogey—For fair and wise legal counsel and for getting my proposal into the hands of Don Pape, publisher and friend.

To the WaterBrook/Shaw team, including Lori Addicott, Laura Barker, Marjorie Barritt, William Bauers, Kirsten Blomquist, Steve Cobb, Stephanie Dickerson, Rita Dotson, Amy Einck, Mark Ford, Kristie Fry, Ron Garcia, Ginia Hairston, Tim Healy, Clark Herrington, Mary Johnson, Molly Johnson,

Jennifer Lonas, Brian McGinley, Leah McMahan, Debbie Mitchell, Maria Parsley, Rod Schumacher, Tim Vanderkolk, Julia Wallace, and Jami Warren— As I know only too well, there is no such thing as a small role in this process. Special thanks to my editor, Elisa Fryling Stanford. Your insight and gentle leading have helped shape this book into what it needed to be.

To Wes Harbour—For friendship and counsel and for introducing me to your incredible wife.

To Susi Harbour—Your willingness to give of yourself has helped to free this former captive.

To Doxology Records: Dan and Sara Posthuma, Marlei Daugherty, Ann-Janette Cormier, and John Newcomer—Your friendship, faith, and flexibility have been welcome blessings this past year.

To the early manuscript readers: Michelle Herrington, Anne McCarthy, Leanne Spencer, and Monique Valdez—Your input was invaluable to me.

To Misty Williams, Sam Chappell, Rick Myers, and Tara Meyer—For your belief in me and your enthusiasm to join the cause.

To my pastors, Jeff Schulte and Lloyd Shadrach, and to so many FBC friends who have become like family to me during this growing process.

To Dana Bianchi, Tina Harris, Beth Jones, and Sherry Parfait—Without your help, I would never have been able to get this thing done and handed in.

To Daren Thomas, film and video producer extraordinaire, and to Velvet Rousseau, Stacie Vining, and Jeni Frankenstein of The Media Collective—Thank you for investing your time and considerable talent to help further the reach of this book.

To those who graciously contributed their thoughts through interviews: Don Durham, Marnie Ferre, Harry Gwirtsman, Vivian Hanson Meehan, Sharon Hersh, Sharlene Hesse-Biber, Gregg Jantz, Nicole Johnson, Alan Schweitzer, and Tracy White—Your perspective has helped reinforce the importance of addressing this issue.

To EMICMG—Your high standards, hard knocks, and strong emphasis on personal growth have all played a role in who I am today and have equipped me immeasurably for the journey I now take. Thank you.

Finally, and most importantly, thank you God for placing in my heart an impossible dream and, in your perfect timing, leading me toward its reality. I am nothing without you.

Foreword

When my daughter asked me to write this foreword, I hoped I would do the book justice. I truly believe that *Life Inside the "Thin" Cage* will touch the lives of thousands of women—and men—in this thin-obsessed culture of ours.

If you have picked up this book, it probably means that you or someone you care for is afraid of never being able to be thin enough. What is "thin" anyway? If you were to poll twenty different people to define what it means to be thin, you would probably get twenty different answers—most of which would lie somewhere between the lowest ideal weight on an accepted weight chart and the distorted media ideal often depicting the threatened condition of the classic anorexic.

Why is being thin so important? Because we equate it with so many personal rights: the right to be respected, the right to be loved, the right to be noticed, the right to be acknowledged at work and appreciated for what we have to offer, the right to wear nice clothes, and even the right to eat what we want, when we want. Oddly, the right to eat is most treasured even when the desired food is only going to be rejected—or purged—anyway.

In a society that rewards thinness and beauty, those who are trapped in an all-encompassing "need" to be thin find that the definition of thin can change from day to day. They are trapped in a cage where dieting, fasting, and binging become a way of life.

Much is written on anorexia and bulimia, and this book addresses these disorders as well. But Constance's main focus is on chronic dieting, which can be just as serious an eating disorder emotionally, physically, and relationally.

Chronic yo-yo dieting is so common and accepted that little is discussed about the grip it has on so many people's lives. We are inundated in the grocery line with pictures of celebrities promoting their latest diet successes and telling us how we, too, can lose unwanted pounds and inches. But no one talks about the fears those movie stars were going through that led them to begin that latest diet. We don't know how many times they go on diets or if they ever really feel satisfied with their new weight. From a physical standpoint, chronic dieting has been related to late-onset diabetes, irritable bowel syndrome, constipation, fatigue, and other serious conditions. Finally, life is often chaotic and depressed for those trapped in chronic dieting. The chronic dieter's world centers on food and eating, so there is little to no priority given to other people. Relationships suffer, leading to feelings of inadequacy, unworthiness, and helplessness.

I know firsthand what it is like being trapped in the thin cage, since for years I struggled in a cage of my own. As a mother, I've also watched Constance fight for freedom from her own thin cage. And as a clinical psychologist, I have seen many clients face similar battles with chronic dieting and disordered eating patterns. For my clients, being thin was the measure of their worthiness. At work, it was their worthiness for respect and acknowledgment. At church, it was their testimony of "God-given" self-discipline. In social and professional circles, it was their ticket to being a part of the group, since surely people who kept their bodies in such good shape were people worth getting to know. For most, achieving a state of thinness offered a lot of attention and flirtatious fun.

To chronic dieters, being thin falsely promises a whole new and fun world. In truth, an unhealthy desire to be thin brings a private shame as they constantly look for ways to eat and not pay the consequences. They try to convince the world they are self-disciplined and living a "normal" lifestyle when in truth they are hiding the reality of their sickness. Many are constantly torn between painful memories of being teased in younger days or feeling as if they were treated like a useless slob when they were heavier. It seems impossible to them that they could ever maintain a healthy "thin" weight without having to live every moment thinking about food! Truly, the obsession with weight and food *is* a cage—with iron bars—and the key to freedom is difficult to find.

This book is written for those who have ever felt trapped in the world of dieting or who have spent too much of their daily lives thinking about food and being thin. It is written with such frankness and intimate detail that you will finally know you're not alone. There is hope! And you do not necessarily have to be "fat" to be free. The key is finding balance in the area of eating and weight control, as well as in all other areas of your life.

Finding balance requires self-acceptance. *Life Inside the "Thin" Cage* will help you find freedom from fear, self-hatred, and shame and will take you on a path to self-discovery and hope. It won't be easy, but it is well worth the struggle. I hope you will dare to take the journey.

—KARYN H. WILLIAMS, Ph.D.

The Undefined Disorder

When I set out to write this book, I struggled for months to come up with the right descriptor for what I wanted to talk about. After wading through ambiguous and confusing terms like *subclinical eating disorder* and *bulimarexia* (the worst of both worlds as one person put it), I finally found a term that seemed to fit what I had so personally struggled with: *chronic dieting.*

In the clinical world (with which I am familiar only through research for this book), chronic dieting would fall into the family of eating disorders referred to as "subclinical," "subthreshold," "partial syndrome," and "EDNOS," all terms used to describe disordered eating not severe enough to fit the classifications of anorexia, bulimia, and binge eating.

That is not to say that those who fit the profile for a subclinical disorder or chronic dieting differ entirely from anorexics, bulimics, or binge eaters, as quite · often many symptoms and patterns are the same. The difference is that not *all* of the criteria for a specific disorder are met, which throws the diagnosis into the black hole of EDNOS (Eating Disorders Not Otherwise Specified)—a catchall term used in the *Diagnostic and Statistical Manual of Mental Disorders* (*DSM-IV*) to refer to disorders falling outside the established types. This means that, by definition, EDNOS remain undefined. Quite the conundrum.

In my mind, it is because they are in this grey, undefined area that subclinical disorders and chronic dieting remain largely undiagnosed and untreated. After all, how can doctors treat a problem that isn't even spelled out in the most complete professional resource of the mental health world? Worse yet, how can sufferers admit their struggle and realize their need for help if they don't even know their problem has a name?

So I've set out to share with you my journey through the compulsive and frustrating world of chronic dieting. The stories that follow are my own as well as those of friends, old and new, who have graciously shared their struggles with me. And while this should not be considered a comprehensive and clinical look at this problem, it represents truth.

May you find hope in these pages.

PART 1

WHEN "THIN" BECOMES A CAGE

I don't have an eating disorder. I just watch what I eat." These were the words I repeated time and again to anyone who suggested that I was overly concerned with weight and dieting. After all, I reasoned, isn't it normal to take pride in maintaining a slim figure?

In Western society today, it is culturally acceptable and even expected that women who want to be successful and respected will be on a never-ending diet. At every turn, we face images of smiling, beautiful, thin people. We can't walk through a shopping mall without realizing that unless we go to extreme measures, we're just not going to be able to stack up against the ideal of beauty that we see hanging in store windows. Even if we don't leave home, an innocent evening in front of the television supplies multiple reminders of the standards we consistently fail to meet.

So we have learned how to force our often rebellious bodies into the crippling corset of conformity. We have exercised, skipped meals, switched to low-fat or no-fat foods, or gradually decreased our overall intake of calories to a point that ensures continued weight loss. As time has gone by, some of us have learned the art of replacing a burger and fries with a Diet Coke and a fruit plate, while others live from diet to diet—a never-ending cycle of feast, famine, elation, and self-loathing.

Even if we are successful at losing a few pounds, it seems we only find new things to dislike about the size and shape of our body. "If I could be just one size smaller," we lament, "then *everything* would be better."

And so the vicious cycle continues, sapping us of time, energy, satisfaction, and self-esteem. Without realizing it, we've become trapped in the "cage" we so lovingly call "thin"—endlessly striving to meet an ideal that seems like the answer to our discontent.

From the undereater to the overeater to the millions in between, everyone's journey to and from the so-called thin cage is undoubtedly different. And yet the view from within is eerily the same.

I invite you to explore the darkest places of one such cage…my own.

Chapter 1

A View from Within

The world goes by my cage and never sees me.

—RANDALL JARRELL (1914–1965), American poet

From my journal, April 2000:

Let me tell you about my life inside the thin cage. It is a dark place with little food, little social interaction, and little freedom. Everything is off-limits. Everything is based on performance. If I don't perform well or look good, then I am not good. I am not allowed to enjoy a piece of cake or a slice of pizza because if I do, tomorrow I will wake up fat. I don't get much social interaction because I scare off any would-be friends out of my fear of letting them get too close to me. I exist on water and a few carefully planned meals every day. And coffee—lots of coffee. And Diet Coke, of course. When I walk into a room, I throw off an intimidating vibe so as to ensure that potential threats to my insecurity (that is, nice people) keep their distance. Other women pick up on the vibe and treat me coldly—something I don't really want but have caused to happen by my behavior.

Daily I complain to my long-suffering husband…"My butt is bigger today, isn't it?" "My stomach didn't look like this last month, did it?" "Are you sure I'm not fat?" "I feel so gross… How can you love me?" It's a wonder he does, but he does.

I'm grouchy all the time and am constantly aware of my cruel nature toward people I wish I could be nicer to.

Since everything is about performance and appearance, a bad hair day can truly ruin me. If my performance ever slips, I am suddenly in the precarious position of losing my value to the world. Going anywhere and meeting anyone requires that I look my best, for people may not like me if they don't think I'm attractive and thin. I have a hard time sleeping at night. More than anything, I'm alone.

How the Story Began

As a young girl, I don't recall ever being unhappy with my body. Even though both of my parents admit to being very weight conscious, I don't remember either of them ever giving me a reason to doubt that my body was just fine. In fact, we didn't even talk about the body types of us kids. Looking back I find this curious, especially because my mother recently told me that she had been quite concerned about my weight when I was a child. As a toddler, I had been significantly chubbier than my older sister, Karen, and Mom was worried that I would end up being fat, as she had been as a young girl.

As I progressed from toddler age to my preteen years, I was still not stick thin, but no one would have called me fat or even chunky. I was "normal."

When I entered my teens, I quickly lost my baby fat and began liking the way I looked in clothes. Like most girls, once in a while I would worry that I had gained a little weight, so I'd go on a diet for a day or so. I've come across some of my diet logs from those days and have been quite amused to read entries such as "ice cream—two scoops," "granola cereal—one bowl," and "one hot dog." Little did I imagine that these foods were loaded with fat and probably were not the best choices when trying to lose weight. But I was blissfully innocent, and my diets were few and far between.

It was during my teen years that I first learned about disordered eating up close and personal. My mother, who had battled her weight since childhood, had been on one diet after another all her life. Following a brief flirtation with bulimia soon after I was born, she spent many years in what she would call an inactive state before once again succumbing to a life-altering eating disorder.

As an educated and curious woman, Mom kept detailed accounts of her struggles in the hope that she could discover the key to freedom from this demon. One day while snooping through her things, I came across several of these journals, and so, long before I would ever struggle with this problem myself, I had the opportunity to enter the mind of someone with an eating disorder. And it scared me.

My First Weight Gain

At the age of sixteen I graduated early from my small Christian high school in Brighton, Michigan, and moved to Dallas to attend a Bible college just south of the big city. Since the school was quite conservative, my parents seemed to feel that I would be fine leaving home so young. I was, of course, quite proud to be on my own; I considered myself to be terribly independent and mature for my age.

Little did I know that I was entering what would prove to be some of the most difficult years of my life. First, there was the fact that three days after registration I was hauled into the dean's office, where I was nervously told, "We had *no idea* you were so young!" and was threatened with being sent home. After some consideration (another sixteen-year-old had been allowed to attend a few years earlier, and my birth date had been clearly stated on my application), it was agreed that I could stay, but under terms of probation until I turned eighteen. To make matters worse, the college's singing group, which had been my entire reason for attending the school, understandably did not want to take a sixteen-year-old girl with them as they toured the country.

With all the turmoil of my freshman year, during that first semester in Dallas, I put on weight for the first time in my life. For some reason, I seemed to be the only one in the dark about the whole Freshman Fifteen phenomenon, a realization that frustrated me greatly once I joined the club. Looking back now I can see that a lot of factors contributed to my weight gain, not the least of which was the fact that I didn't know the first thing about cooking. With a few dollars in my pocket, I headed out to buy whatever was easy, cheap, and different from the menu I had grown up with. Add to this the stress of adjusting to living in an adult world, and eating took on new meaning and purpose for me.

Having never worried about my weight before, it didn't strike me that what (and how much) I was eating might turn into unwanted weight gain. It wasn't until a couple of months later that I realized I was in trouble. I was trying on clothes at The Limited when suddenly my reflection in the three-way mirror caused me to recoil in horror. "What's *that?*" I gasped. It appeared that I had some extra growth happening around my middle. As I investigated more closely, turning this way and that, I realized with shock and terror that I seemed to be growing an extra butt, just above where my current one had once resided in beauty and, most important, solitude. *What is happening?* I cried. It took me a little while to understand the problem—I was gaining weight. Still in denial, I headed for my apartment to weigh myself. The scale confirmed what the mirror had jeeringly suggested: I had gained about fifteen pounds.

I was devastated. Here I was, facing the fact that life had unexpectedly turned me on my ear in nearly every way imaginable. And with just a few weeks to go before Christmas vacation, I panicked. *I can't go home like this,* I thought. *What will they all think of me?* I just couldn't imagine having nothing positive to report to my family. Nothing had gone right so far, and now I felt fat for the first time in my life.

So I did what any logical girl does. I headed for the diet books and frantically searched for one that promised quick results. Then a friend told me about her success with a grapefruit diet, and I decided that this might be just the ticket. After all, I had a few weeks, and with this diet you were supposed to lose ten pounds in two weeks. Anxiously, I peeled my first grapefruit, determined to stick it out until I reached my goal. "I like grapefruit," I told myself.

After about a day of this, my insides were on fire, and even my intense fear of fat wasn't strong enough to keep me on my regimen. So I ate something, which triggered several days of binging and only made matters worse. Suffice it to say, I was still carrying the extra unwanted pounds when I walked off the plane to meet my family for the holiday season. I felt like a failure. I felt fat. I felt unattractive. I felt as though I had lost my edge. And I vowed to do something about it.

Flirting with the Dark Side

Looking back I realize that no one even noticed my weight gain that Christmas. I can remember making excuses about it, but no one seemed concerned except me. I wish I could have believed them, but I didn't. I knew I liked being slim, and the idea of losing that status terrified me.

After the holidays I felt even worse. I had pigged out on all the Christmas goodies and was now more than fifteen pounds over my college-entry weight—a number that had been indelibly marked in my brain as the goal I had to attain at any cost.

When I arrived back on campus, I wasn't sure what to do. I wanted the weight to be gone as unexpectedly as it had arrived, but I was quickly coming to understand that I was going to have to fight for this change. I yo-yoed for several months—a typical pattern of success, failure, success. Even so, by the end of the school year I was feeling pretty good, having lost about half of the initial weight I had gained. But my struggles were far from over.

That summer I moved in with my friends Mike and D'Onna who lived in North Dallas. One day, intent on proving my value to the household, I worked laboriously for about seven hours in the hot Texas sun, removing twigs, branches, and tangled underbrush from the long-neglected pool area. Little did I know that the "weeds" I was pulling were actually poison oak! The next day, puffy-faced and wheezing, I was hauled into the emergency room, where I was prescribed prednisone (a steroid) to bring the intense rash under control. When I got back from the hospital, I popped the pills and did my usual weigh-in. The scale confirmed that my efforts were paying off: I had lost another pound. Just eight more to go and I would be at my precollege weight!

That night I felt I deserved to eat. I was miserable from my rash and had only had a salad for lunch, so I reasoned that it would be okay to eat just a little. Cautiously, I ate one of D'Onna's famous chocolate-chip cookies, telling myself, "This is all you get!" when suddenly my brain started buzzing. An overwhelming desire for food seemed to take control of me, and I headed for the well-stocked pantry to survey my options. By the end of the evening, I had eaten so much that my stomach ached. Frustrated at my lack of self-control and scared that all my efforts were now wasted, I clicked into excuse mode, telling myself that since I had already blown it, I may as well make the most of the weekend.

On Monday, resolved to get back on the program, I nervously stepped onto the scale, and my deepest fears were confirmed: *Oh no! I had gained ten pounds! It didn't seem possible! Had I really eaten that much?*

What I didn't realize at the time was that the prednisone was making me retain water, which had a significant impact on the numbers I saw on the scale. This alarming increase totally freaked me out and triggered a binge that seemed to continue for the rest of the summer.

Anorexia

At the end of the summer, I reentered college at my heaviest weight so far. I was miserable and somehow found the determination to stop binging. It was then that I entered into anorexia for the first time.

During my third semester at school, I ate only Malt-O-Meal, three times a day. Each time it had to be cooked in the same pot, eaten with the same spoon, and sweetened with just two packets of Equal. I didn't realize it at the time, but I was behaving like a textbook anorexic. Had I been aware of the danger of my actions though, I wouldn't have cared—I was now losing weight rapidly. By Christmas, I was exactly at my precollege weight, though my body seemed to look different somehow. I soon realized that my natural muscle tone had been replaced with fatty cellulite as a result of the binging and rapid weight loss. This frustrated me, but I consoled myself, thinking that if I could lose just a little more, I'd once again be happy with my body.

This active anorexic stage was a tough one. I became incredibly isolated. I could not bring myself to make eye contact with others, and I avoided the social interaction I so desperately needed. I was chronically fatigued, which caused me to take naps on the job, where I worked for the on-campus painting department. (No one found out, thankfully, though my boss did wonder why it took so long for me to complete projects.)

I grew content in my starvation, proud to see my body shrink. I even saw it as a positive side effect that I no longer had periods. *How nice not to have to bother with that,* I thought. But even though I was happy with my weight loss, I was still unhappy with my body. That Christmas my family was a little concerned. My weight had plummeted considerably since my last visit. At mealtimes I would just push food around on the plate; I even bought my own Malt-O-Meal so I could continue my routine. It's strange to me now that no one really got in my face about it—though I don't know if it would have done any good anyway.

Bulimia

A few months after Christmas, I entered the break room between classes and passed by the doughnut table. *Those look so good,* I thought to myself, as I did nearly every day. *Hmmm, I wonder if I could have just one? After all, I have lost a significant amount of weight, and it wouldn't even hurt me if I gained a pound—I could just lose it again.*

So I reasoned myself into purchasing the heavenly treat. As I ate it, my pleasure was immense. *See,* I told myself. *You deserve this. You can handle this.* My taste buds seemed to pop in delight at the unexpected flavor. I ate faster and faster, and then the sugar hit my brain, a rush more intense than anything I had experienced before. I was energized. I was scared. I wanted another doughnut. I needed it *NOW.*

So I purchased another, and this time I paced myself. *You don't want to lose all the progress you've made, do you?* the voice inside my head reminded me. I finished the doughnut and walked away, proud of myself for having the discipline to eat just two. *I'll make up for it by skipping dinner tonight.* And I did.

A few days later it was my roommate's birthday. Ever since eating those doughnuts, all I could think about were sweets, which is probably why I decided to make some brownies for her birthday. I bought the most delectable brownie mix I could find and set off for home to bake them.

As I mixed the ingredients, I toyed with the idea of giving myself just a little taste. Convinced I could handle it, I stuck my finger in the bowl and gave it a lick. Wow! The batter was so good. *But you can't eat more,* I told myself and dutifully put the brownies in the oven to bake. When they came out, I told myself

I should try just one to make sure that they were done. It was delicious. *Just one more,* I thought as I wolfed another down.

Before I knew what was happening, I had eaten half the pan. Now I was really concerned. I knew that this was not good, especially coming on the heels of my forbidden doughnuts from the other day. In slowly rising terror, I considered my options and decided that throwing up was probably my best bet. *Quick, easy, and convenient,* I thought. So I headed to the toilet and stuck my finger down my throat. Nothing happened. I didn't seem to have the right technique. Stubbornly I continued trying until it finally worked. As the brownies came up, images of my mother's journals flashed into my mind, and chillingly I realized I was on the threshold of wreaking incredible havoc in my life. This was quite sobering.

My flirtation with purging did not last long. Wise to the inherent danger, I never let myself get good at throwing up. I tried laxatives a few times, but they made me so sick that I just couldn't take it. The sugar from my frequent overeating was taking its toll on me though, and I no longer had the power to resist the binges that were happening with alarming regularity.

The Binge-Starve Cycle

Once I was determined not to throw up or use laxatives, the only way to compensate for my binges was to try to offset them with periods of restraint. This was only slightly less traumatic a lifestyle than purging had been, as I constantly felt trapped in a vicious cycle of either eating too much or not enough. There is no way to effectively lose weight in this state, and I soon found myself growing even heavier than I had been the summer before. "When will this cycle stop?" I cried out. I even called the mother of a friend of mine who had been admitted to a treatment facility. As I cried on the phone with her, I found myself wishing I could be checked in someplace where someone would just take all the food away so I couldn't hurt myself anymore. But I didn't have the funds for this, and I didn't want to delay graduating from college, so I didn't pursue it.

For over a year I continued this type of eating. I settled in at about twenty-eight pounds heavier than I wished to be and lingered there for a while. I somehow stopped the more intense binging but continued eating more than I needed to.

Later that year I was finally invited to join my school's singing group and left on a three-month tour. I wasn't binging anymore, but I hated my body. I felt very heavy in the uniform I wore on stage, and I was constantly comparing myself to other thinner girls. I also grew increasingly frustrated by the lack of control I had over what I ate. Since I didn't have any money with which to buy my own food, I was limited to the meals that were provided for us. These were usually high in fat—pizza, lasagna, fried chicken. Somewhere along the way I resigned myself to the fact that I couldn't get away from the food, and I just went for broke, figuring I'd fix the problem when I finally returned home.

Then one day on tour, I reached a turning point. I forced myself to look in the mirror and face the truth about my body. Painfully, I turned myself so that I could see every angle. I was devastated. I felt completely trapped in a body that looked increasingly different than it had just a year earlier. This body wasn't me. I knew that I needed to cut back on the amounts I was eating. I decided that if I did something about it, I would never have to look any larger than I did at this moment.

It was then that I decided to start dieting, gradually, one meal at a time. *Why rush?* I told myself. *It's never worked before.*

And as I finally learned how to control my appetite, I wandered into what became for me a normal way of life—constant or chronic dieting.

When Dieting Turns Chronic

Dieting isn't a phase for me. It's a lifestyle.

—MELANIE, age thirty-seven

Who would have imagined that being disciplined at dieting would actually be a bad thing? I mean, to be able to resist nachos and choose grilled chicken instead—that's a good thing, right? And what could be wrong with learning how to control ourselves enough to just leave that huge helping of cake on the plate? Isn't this what we're all supposed to strive for?

As with all things, healthy eating requires a balance in such areas as what we eat, when we eat, and how much we eat, and even in our view of the role food should play in our life. The question I finally had to ask myself was "Am I balanced when it comes to eating and weight?" And the answer was unequivocally no.

I had become so consumed with the fear of gaining weight that I was on an endless and unforgiving diet. Following my initial weight loss after I graduated, I remained on this diet even though I was thin. Did I need to be on a diet? No. I would have been reasonably thin anyway, without all the grief. But I didn't know that. All I knew was that if I dared to eat just one forbidden bite, all would be lost, and I'd slip back into the frustrating weight gain I had experienced in college.

At the Crossroads

It was Christmas of 1998. My husband and I were in Michigan visiting my family for the holidays. It was a quick visit, with the ever-present demands of work waiting for us upon our return home. On the last day of our visit, my father took me to breakfast at one of his favorite hole-in-the-wall restaurants in the small town of Brighton where I grew up. I ordered a poached egg, dry toast, and coffee. Everything was going along just fine until he looked me in the eye for a moment. I knew what was coming.

"I'm concerned about you," he began. "You're too thin."

"Dad," I complained, "you're always picking on me. I don't have an eating disorder. I know all about what those are from watching Mom's struggle with bulimia and anorexia. I may have had a problem for a couple of years, but now I'm just careful about what I eat. I don't want to get fat, but I'm not anorexic."

"Con, you are too thin. What if you were to get into a car accident and be physically injured? You wouldn't have the energy to fight back! You have no meat on your bones left to lose."

"I don't agree, Dad," I replied. "I've been to the doctor several times this year for various little things, and every time I go she gives me a clean bill of health."

"Have you told her how you eat?" he asked.

I considered this carefully. "I guess not," I admitted. "If it will make you happy, I'll go again, tell her how I'm eating, and see what she has to say. But trust me, I don't have an eating disorder. I just enjoy being a little thin. I don't want to waste away to nothing; I just like the way clothes look on me when I'm this thin."

True to my promise, I made an appointment with my doctor, and a few weeks later, I was sitting in her office, resolved to tell her exactly how I had been living.

"I'm here because I think I might not be eating quite right," I said. I proceeded to tell her that sometimes if I thought I ate too much at lunch, I'd just skip dinner. Or if I ate too much one day, I might not eat the next day, just to make up for it. But then I might eat pizza, or something else normal, so you see, I wasn't an anorexic, because an anorexic wouldn't touch a piece of pizza.

She wrote all this down in my file and then asked me, "Do you want to live to be a skinny, brittle old lady?" It didn't sound all that bad to me. Better to be skinny than fat, right?

She then proceeded to take my blood pressure and do a number of tests, including blood work and even an EKG. That was a little weird—I had never had to have one of those done before. I mean, really, I was only twenty-seven. I smiled with satisfaction as all of the blood tests again came back normal. I was healthy after all, just as I thought. My little weight control plan couldn't be all that bad.

Which is why a shock went through me when I read the diagnosis the doctor wrote on the bottom of my little pink slip: anorexia.

Anorexia? I thought anorexia meant starving day after day, eating a grape and a lettuce leaf and calling it a meal, missing periods, growing lanugo (body hair), and eventually being hospitalized, dying a death of refusal of food!

I paid my ten-dollar copay and wandered down the steps to my car. Confused, dazed, and emotionally stripped, I got into the car and just sat there for a few moments. The voices began to swirl in my head: *Anorexia... You have to admit there's a problem... I guess I have been a little preoccupied with this weight thing... Oh God, this is a moment of decision.* And then the tears came. I'm not totally sure what I was crying about, but I know that I was scared. Scared to admit that I had a problem. Scared that everyone else had known it all along and I had somehow been blind to it. Scared that everyone was going to think I was a loser. Scared that I had let myself get to this point.

It was an incredibly pivotal moment for me.

Subclinical Eating Disorders and the EDNOS Category

As I sat in my car on that rainy January day in 1999, I considered my options. I could choose to throw out the diagnosis of anorexia, since, having read through my mother's medical books, I knew that I no longer fit all the criteria (though I realized that I was highly anorexic in my thinking). Or, even though anorexia wasn't the most accurate diagnosis, I could accept it as a name for my behavior and place my focus on trying to deal with what was a very real problem in my life: an unhealthy obsession with weight. By God's providence, this is what I chose.

As I came to a healthier place in my approach to eating and food, it became clear to me that this disorder of mine lacked a proper name. This frustrated me. Not only did I not want to be called anorexic if I didn't fully fit the profile, but when I finally did begin to seek counseling for my problem, no one seemed to know what to do with me. I was no longer an active anorexic, and I definitely wasn't practicing bulimia or even binge eating, but it seemed that therapists were looking for me to be one extreme or the other. One psychologist even put me on Prozac and recommended Rapid Eye Movement therapy. I was growing increasingly disturbed with the fact that no one seemed to understand exactly what I was facing. How was I supposed to get help if people didn't "get" the problem?

Fast-forward to Christmas of 2000. I was in Virginia visiting my mother and told her about the book I wanted to write. I explained my belief that there is a whole group of women and men who might not fit all the criteria for anorexia, bulimia, or binge eating, but who have a unique and very real problem that needs to be addressed. In our conversation I referred to it as an "in-between" disorder.

She copied off for me some pages from the *Diagnostic and Statistical Manual of Mental Disorders (DSM-IV),* a reference manual for professionals who work with mental disorders of all types. Sandwiched between several pages of information on anorexia, bulimia, overeating, and binge-eating disorders, I discovered a short little segment termed EDNOS (Eating Disorders Not Otherwise Specified).

Finally! In these paragraphs, I found the exact problem I was struggling with. Those who have EDNOS—also called subclinical or subthreshold disorders—fit part but not all of the profiles of the better-known problems. For example, in my case I had several anorexic behaviors but hadn't been missing any periods, which I took as a clear sign that I was not clinically anorexic.

Other disordered eaters might be borderline bulimics or binge eaters, but since they don't fit all the criteria, they feel misunderstood and wrongly labeled. But the EDNOS category provides a home for us. If someone had talked to me about this before, I probably would have been more willing to admit that I had a problem.

To better understand EDNOS, it is helpful to think of eating habits as being on a continuum. At one end of the continuum are the more extreme forms of eating disorders, such as anorexia, bulimia, and binge eating. On the other end is healthy eating. Between these points are unhealthy behaviors that, while not considered extreme, can significantly affect the way we live our lives. In my case,

I bounced from one end of the continuum to the other, finally ending up in the EDNOS category. Some people start in this category only to move on to more dangerous behaviors. Others never reach the behavioral extremes but live in a never-ending nightmare of the in-between, obsessed with weight, and preoccupied with looking a certain way.

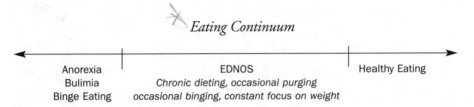

Eating Continuum

| Anorexia
Bulimia
Binge Eating | EDNOS
Chronic dieting, occasional purging
occasional binging, constant focus on weight | Healthy Eating |

You Don't Have to Be Skinny to Be Weight Obsessed

One of the most common misconceptions about chronic dieters is that we are all skinny. The fact is, while some chronic dieters have indeed reached and maintained a weight that is in the low range, many people of average or higher weight also struggle with the same unhealthy obsession to be thin.

Consider Jolene. She is a size 11/12. At every meal she beats herself up, thinking, *Oh no! I just finished everything on my plate. Everyone else must think I'm a pig. They all know I need to lose ten pounds. Oh, I just wish I had ordered a salad instead. Now I'm going to have to skip dinner.* Meanwhile, Jolene's friends around the table have no clue that she wrestles with this demon daily. They think to themselves, *Must be nice to be able to eat everything on your plate.* They assume that because Jolene is a "regular" size, she does not worry about her weight. They figure that she has managed to feel comfortable with the fact that she's never going to be a petite girl. They'd be shocked to hear the dialogue running through her mind at every meal.

I was recently reminded of this paradox when talking with a very attractive woman of average weight. We were discussing this book, specifically some of the thought patterns I was writing about, and I made the comment, "Of course this probably sounds strange to you, since you probably haven't struggled with eating."

She looked back at me in surprise, "Oh, I think about it all the time. I've been considering going on Slim-Fast so I can lose some weight. I just feel so fat!"

She proceeded to tell me how she skips meals frequently and tries to eat fat-free foods whenever she can, but even with her efforts she just can't seem to lose weight. Because she seemed to me to be an average size, I had just assumed that she wasn't caught in the thin cage. But I've learned that you don't have to be skinny to be ruled by an obsession to be thin.

An Unexpected Struggle

I've often been frustrated by those who, through lack of understanding, say, "You got yourself into this situation; now just get yourself out." The point they're missing is that we never intended to be "in this situation." Now finding our way out is going to be difficult for many reasons, not the least of which is that being thin is often rewarded in our culture. Leanne Spencer, a licensed professional counselor, makes the following comparison:

> [Telling a weight-obsessed woman to stop obsessing] is like telling a drug dealer, who makes five thousand a week selling crack and heroin, to stop for the betterment of the community. He drives a Porsche, buys anything he wants, and has money to spare. As long as he perceives status as a direct result of his efforts, he has little reason to quit. In the same manner, women get attention for looking good and wearing hip-hugger jeans to showcase their thin, flat, sunken-in stomachs.[1]

Just as in the case of the drug dealer, our obsession has its dangers. Spencer adds,

> The problem is that what seems like a "good thing" and appears to be mere "self-discipline" is actually a ritual that begins to deny life and crush our spirits. Instead of being healthy, we are an object that retains value from being "perfect" or without mark. Our preciousness is no longer defined by the beauty of our soul or the standing of our spirit. We are the looks we draw.[2]

And so we find ourselves in a confusing, unnamed, misunderstood cage of wanting to be someone other than who we are. Thin is both the adversary we wrestle with and our ideal identity. And since we are often hesitant to admit the strength of our obsession, we are left unaware that many others struggle in the same way we do.

Just How Big a Problem Is It?

In the absence of hard data, Anorexia Nervosa and Related Eating Disorders Inc. (ANRED) states, "We can only guess at the vast numbers of people who have sub-clinical or threshold eating disorders."[3] Christopher Fairburn and Terence Wilson, authors of *Binge Eating: Nature, Assessment and Treatment,* add, "The [EDNOS] category tends to get overlooked despite common clinical experience that a sizable proportion of patients belong to it."[4] To get a more accurate picture of the prevalence of subclinical disorders, consider the following diagram:

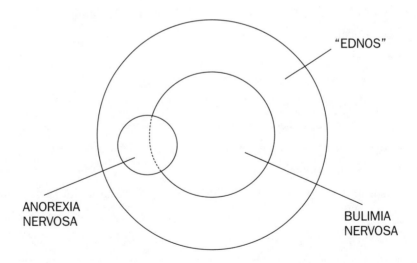

A schematic representation of the relationship between the diagnosis anorexia nervosa, bulimia nervosa, and eating disorders not otherwise specified (EDNOS). From Binge Eating: Nature, Assessment and Treatment; © 1993 by Christopher G. Fairburn and G. Terence Wilson. Reprinted by permission.

You can imagine my excitement when I came across this diagram while doing research for this book. Finally, someone was putting the problem into perspective. As you can see, the circles representing anorexia and bulimia overlap, indicating a small but significant group of people who suffer with a combination of the two. Surrounding both of them is the much larger area of EDNOS—confirmation that we exist!

Indeed, as I began interviewing counselors and therapists, it was repeatedly confirmed: Many more women struggle with chronic dieting and nonextreme eating disorders than with full-blown eating disorders.

Sharon Hersh, author of *"Mom, I Feel Fat!"* tells me, "In my practice, if one out of four has a diagnosable eating disorder, two out of the other three have a subclinical disorder."[5] Leanne Spencer puts it this way:

> If we had an effective, true environment in which to get women to
> respond honestly about body perception, eating habits, diet practices,
> and obsessions with food, we would see a very high percentage that fit
> the EDNOS category. If forced to guess, I would say that 85 percent
> of women have distorted views about weight, and 70 percent of those
> progress to subclinical behaviors.[6]

In certain environments, the problem seems especially concentrated. According to research done by Dr. Alan Schwitzer and his colleagues at Old Dominion University in Virginia, college campuses are particularly dense breeding grounds for disordered eating. Between 25 and 40 percent of women on college campuses struggle with unhealthy attitudes toward eating and weight. And yet only 6 percent would be considered clinically anorexic or bulimic, indicating that a large percentage of students might not be getting help for their problem. Because of this, Dr. Schwitzer tells me, "Resources would be much better spent on mid-disorders. Refer out the more extreme cases... Subclinical problems affect more people."[7]

Within the athletic community, where high value is placed upon form and fitness, subclinical disorders are rampant. As one researcher notes, "The prevalence of sub-clinical eating disorders exceeds that of clinical eating disorders among female athletes."[8] Since people of all ages participate in sports, children and adolescents, as well as adult men and women, are feeling the pressure to be lean.

Perhaps a final test of the breadth of this problem is to consider how many other people you know who are constantly obsessing about their weight and feel the need to diet continually. According to a study done in 2000, nearly 65 million American women are on a diet on any given day. Of these, 35 percent—more than *22 million* women—progress to pathological dieting.[9] And these figures don't take into account the millions of men who also struggle. When considering these statistics, we can't overlook the fact that this little-discussed problem has quietly claimed an unhealthy role in the lives of millions of people.

Why Isn't Anyone Talking About It?

When we are presented with the staggering numbers of those struggling with subclinical forms of disordered eating, it's only natural to wonder why we haven't really heard anyone talking about this problem. Unfortunately, in a culture that thrives on extremes, from ultrathin models to supersize meals, nonextreme forms of disordered eating are easy to overlook and even excuse.

A Cultural Mandate

For many, chronic dieting and subclinical eating disorders are a logical and accepted response to our most pervasive cultural mandate: "You must be thin and beautiful if you want to be successful in life." And while most of us can't do much to improve upon our God-given looks, we see the size of our bodies as negotiable...something we can surely change. Because of this, it has become socially acceptable, and even expected, that we do whatever it takes to bring our "disobedient" weight under control.

And everyone's in on it. It seems that every third commercial on television is peddling methods and products to help us in our quest—Slim-Fast, Metabolife, Ab Rollers, even too-good-to-be-true solutions such as electric pulse machines, supposedly designed to give us a workout while we sit on our butts eating ice cream. For those who can afford a more radical approach, tummy tucks and liposuction are available—never mind the horror stories we've all heard or the fact that weight lost through medical means is often regained.[10]

We see those who are successful at losing weight applauded, praised, and hailed as the disciplined and attractive people we all wish to be. Is it any wonder, then, that many of us—overweight, underweight, and in-between—have fallen into a pattern of chronic dieting as we strive to fit the "thin is beautiful" ideal?

Consider these facts:

- Three-quarters of women within normal weight limits feel too fat, desiring on average to weigh only slightly more than anorexics.[11]
- The weight of many Miss America winners classifies them as under-nourished.[12]
- Most fashion models are thinner than 98 percent of American women.[13]
- Eighty percent of American women are dissatisfied with their appearance.[14]
- When surveyed, children say they'd prefer being handicapped to being fat.[15]
- Ninety-five percent of dieters suffer from weight cycling (gaining and losing weight).[16]
- Actresses wearing a size 4 are told that they are fat by Hollywood executives.[17]

This is just a tiny snapshot of some of the bars that have made up our cage. Of course, our media-saturated culture is not going anywhere, and we certainly have to contend with being residents of it. But it is important to realize we have a choice whether to buy into the lie that being thin is the ultimate achievement. Leanne Spencer puts it this way,

> We have come to believe that being thin is the one thing that will fulfill us in life. The ironic part is that once we've achieved thinness through our unhealthy obsessions, we are less fulfilled and more incomplete than when we weighed more.[18]

But it isn't just our culture that has become numb to our plight. Even the medical community at large seems to have turned a deaf ear to the emerging cries for help.

Not a "Significant" Medical Problem

Those who try to fight the culture and seek help for their unhealthy eating practices often discover that few medical professionals seem to appreciate the seriousness of their condition. In exploring this dilemma, I found several reasons for this apparent lack of concern.

First, most therapists would agree that eating disorders are exceedingly complicated, with no single cause or cure. Add to that the billions of dollars spent on research and the treatment of 8 to 10 million Americans reported to struggle with more extreme and even fatal forms of disordered eating, and we already have a significant problem requiring attention.

Is it any surprise, then, that we who struggle with less life-threatening forms of weight control are paid little heed by the medical, clinical, and counseling communities? After all, these professionals have been charged with helping those who could actually die as a result of their battles with eating. In this context, chronic dieting and other subclinical disorders could easily be viewed as mere inconveniences rather than the significant problems they are.

A second reason is the somewhat ambiguous nature of the EDNOS category. As Dr. Harry Gwirtsman, associate professor of psychiatry at Vanderbilt University says, "EDNOS is a wastebasket term. Basically, everything that doesn't conform to something that can be pigeonholed gets tossed in the 'bin.'"[19]

The trouble with this so-called bin is that, as we discussed earlier in this chapter, eating behaviors occur on a continuum, with several points between normal and unhealthy. Lumping all of these behaviors together makes them very difficult to treat individually. Sharlene Hesse-Biber, professor of sociology at Boston College and author of a report on continuum versus noncontinuum approaches,[20] tells me, "Subclinical issues are very important…but we don't have the sensitivity in our measures to effectively get at the pain of these women."[21]

Since therapists don't have a standardized eating continuum to which they can refer, many skip over the EDNOS category altogether and diagnose eating behaviors as being either "normal" or "sick," rather than allowing for the many points in-between. This is also problematic. As Hesse-Biber explains,

Therapists who do not look at eating as being on a continuum will declare patients to be "normal" as soon as they no longer fit the parameters for the clinical disorders. But doing so masks the problem, as their behavior should actually be considered to be in a "grey" category.[22]

Because of these and other realities, many insurers will not reimburse for the Not-Otherwise-Specified category. This is unfortunate because increasing evidence indicates that untreated subclinical disorders often lead to more fullblown syndromes. It is generally agreed that if funding and information were available during the earlier phases of such disorders, fewer people would end up being anorexic or bulimic. For example, one researcher states, "Patients with bulimia nervosa almost invariably report that they developed their binge-purge eating behaviors following a prolonged period of severe dieting."[23]

While it is not the purpose of this book to find fault with our medical and insurance systems, it is important to understand that the lack of focus placed on this problem by the professional community is reinforced by the fact that insurance companies won't even acknowledge the problem exists. It is hard to say which has more influence over the other, but I often wonder what would happen if the millions of chronic dieters started showing up in therapists' offices.

The truth is, millions of nonextreme disordered eaters are suffering silently with significant issues that need to be addressed. We'll explore many of these issues in the following chapters.

The Thought Process

My thoughts were like unbridled children, grown too headstrong for their mother.

—CRESSIDA, in Shakespeare's *Troilus and Cressida*

For the nonextreme, disordered eater, much of our battle is evidenced only in our mind, invisible to others and blindly accepted by ourself. So as I began to more carefully consider the way I had been living for the previous ten years, I became increasingly aware of how strange and powerful my thought processes had become.

Mind Games

In the sections that follow, we'll see how varied, specific, and destructive our thoughts can be when we place an unhealthy emphasis on dieting and weight control.

"Will My Clothes Still Fit Me Today?"

One of the most frustrating things about disordered eating is the warped body image that makes us think that, although our jeans fit yesterday, surely they won't fit today, since we ate an extra serving at dinner last night. I would often go days avoiding certain clothes (pants, usually), convinced that I had some-how—overnight—grown a size bigger. My husband used to laugh at the illogi-cal nature of my thinking. Even so, I would always be surprised when, after finally daring to try the clothes on, they not only fit but were even a little looser as a result of the paranoia-induced restricted eating of the previous few days. What a maddening yo-yo! My friend has what she calls "safe" clothes for these days—loose-fitting clothes that keep her from feeling fat.

"The Mirror Is My Enemy"

It's no secret that those of us who struggle with eating and weight issues experience an ongoing war with the mirror. For most of my adult life I avoided it almost entirely, intent to focus only on its reflection of my face and refusing to look down unless I was fully clothed. Unfortunately, this left the true picture of my body to my imagination (a dangerous thing to do, considering).

I have a friend in Seattle who is just the opposite—she can't walk by the mirror without standing sideways, sticking out her stomach, and walking away having confirmed to herself what a loser she is for having a belly at all. The interesting thing is that this woman holds a high position at a very reputable company and is obviously a capable and talented individual—yet the flatness of her stomach has become the daily gauge of her value. The problem with relying on mirrors for our measure of self-worth is that we have turned the beauty of our own unique reflection into an opportunity to judge ourselves against the airbrushed images we see in the media.

"Oh, Those Scales"

I am not a huge fan of frequent weighing. Over the years I've seen this practice cause much more harm than good in people's lives. Thankfully, even while I struggled through many years of weight obsession, I always somehow had the common sense to avoid scales. I'm reminded of the wisdom of this each time I have to go to the doctor and get on the scale. Following visits when the number on the scale went up, I would agonize to my husband, "Surely I could allow two pounds for these shoes I was wearing, and another for these clothes, which means I didn't really gain that much weight…"

Doctor visits increased when I was pregnant, and while I had truly made progress in my thoughts about eating—and even in spite of my concern for my unborn child—I was still inclined to restrict my diet a little the week before seeing the doctor to make sure the scale tipped in my favor.

Often, women with disordered eating will get on the scale backward out of fear of how they might react to its judgment. I can relate to this. Scales often play into a dangerous thought process if we are inclined to obsess about the numbers we see.

Warped Body Image

Many of us who obsess about our weight have an image of ourselves that is inconsistent with the "us" that others see. A common therapy for eating-disorder sufferers called "body tracings" addresses this problem. During this exercise, the person is instructed to draw a life-size outline of how big she thinks her body is. She is then instructed to position herself against the drawing. In most cases, the outline of the drawing is several sizes larger than she really is, illustrating that what we *think* we look like and what we *actually* look like are generally two very different things. I was often reminded of this when I would point out an actress on television or a girl in the mall and say to my husband, "Wow, she's so very thin," to which he'd usually reply, "Honey, she is no thinner than you." He wasn't trying to make me feel good; he was just being honest. But of course, I couldn't imagine that I actually looked that thin. My sense of body size had become warped through years of obsessive living.

"What Size Am I?"

I used to believe that each time I went clothes shopping, I should have achieved a smaller size than the last time. Of course, once you reach the lower sizes, you run out of goals, especially if you're of slightly above-average height. But shrinking ever smaller became my obsession. Luckily, my budget didn't allow for frequent clothes shopping, or I would have tied myself up in knots worrying about this.

Hunger: Friend or Foe?

I used to think that I felt my best when I went to bed with an empty stomach. Not only did I think that it was good for my stomach to be empty, but I also took certain comfort in actually feeling hunger pangs as I drifted off into a fitful sleep. I liked the way my thin arms rested against my bony hips—somehow

I felt strong by being so weak. Like many who struggle with disordered eating, I believed that a full stomach would expose my true weakness because I had eaten too much.

Others have the opposite feeling about hunger. During her disorder, my mom actually suffered from a terrible fear of feeling hunger because such feelings would almost certainly send her into a binge. Because of the heightened importance those of us in an eating-disordered state place on hunger, it often loses its natural purpose.

Thin Equals Control Equals Power!

While I believe control to be just one of many factors in an eating disorder, it is definitely one that bears some attention. Until recently I worked in the marketing department of a record company in Nashville. I remember feeling that as long as I was the thinnest person in the boardroom, I had made a very important statement of control, which made me feel more powerful. Exercising this element of control seemed even more important to me in that setting because, as is often the case in corporate environments, one rarely feels entirely confident of one's own value on a consistent basis. Perhaps I thought that as long as I could control the "thin" thing, I would be perceived as powerful and valuable, and I would be assured that, on some level, my supervisors had confidence in me.

"Look at Me! I Am Thin!"

While some of us view weight loss as a way to become smaller and smaller, thus fading from public notice, many of us actually revel in our accomplishment and wish to make sure that everyone else does too. I remember how in my ultrathin days I would hold my head high, enjoying the admiring looks of men and even secretly being satisfied when I noticed the jealous glances of other women less "lucky" than I was. It's a strange state because at the very moment that I was enjoying the attention I received, my own insecurities only seemed to loom larger. For many of us, it's as if we need those approving glances and the attention from others to fill what has become an emotionally barren "bank account." Unfortunately, the more attention we get, the more we need, until we're trapped in a vicious cycle.

"I Am Invincible!"

For those of us who learn to master our bodies through dieting or exercise, there comes a point when we begin to feel invincible, as though no one and nothing can get in our way. We think that if we can just reach or maintain a certain weight, we will be indestructible. It's ironic that even though we feel invincible, we are actually quite powerless and are on our way to becoming crippled—which is one of the cruelest jokes of this disorder.

Obsessive Checking of Body Parts

One of the most common rituals of someone who suffers from a fear-of-fat disorder is the obsessive checking of certain body parts. In my anorexic phase, I remember how pleased I was to realize that I'd lost so much weight that my breasts had nearly disappeared. I would often check to make sure they stayed small as confirmation that I was not getting fat anywhere else. Other obsessions over the years included jutting hips and the number of bones I could count between my clavicle bones and the top of my breasts. I've also read about some women who fixate on the amount of ITC (inner thigh clearance) they have; that is, how closely their thighs are touching (or not) when they stand in front of the mirror. Others focus on the size of their belly or some other body part they think indicates fat, or failure, which brings us to our next problem.

"But My Face Is Fat!"

The other day my sister, Karen, asked me if I thought women with rounder faces might struggle more with thinking they need to lose weight. My immediate response was "Yes, of course!" I hadn't really thought about it lately, but this has always been a trigger for me. While my sister has been blessed with one of those perfect ovals that don't seem to change much, even if her weight significantly increases, I happen to have the type of face that shows weight gain almost immediately. Because of this, I am always a little paranoid about gaining weight out of a fear that my face will become fat.

Even if you don't have a round face, most of us have at least one body part that seems fatter to us than other body parts. We often use this fattest area to gauge whether we have lost enough weight. The problem with doing this is that sometimes, in our efforts to get our naturally muscular arms or fuller thighs under control, we starve our whole body to the extent that we still look disproportionate.

"I Must Not Take Up Too Much Space"

This thought pattern must originate from the fear of rejection—the I-must-not-be-a-burden message that so many of us learn in different ways as children. As I delved into my own thought processes, I realized that I thought it important, even essential, that I not take up what I considered to be too much space. If I could just take a little space, no one would ever think I was in the way. For instance, when I would travel in a car with a large number of people, I would feel good knowing that I was small enough not to take up very much space on the seat. This particular pattern of thinking was very instrumental in pushing me to want to shrink smaller and smaller.

Nonstop Distraction and Constant Comparison

Later in this book we're going to discuss the "message of the tapes": those voices that run nonstop through the mind of someone obsessed with food, dieting, and weight. It is because of these tapes that we find ourselves continually distracted. I can recall whole conversations passing me by while I sat detached, engrossed in determining whether I was on track for the day, or whether I had eaten too much at lunch. Social events that should have been fun were spent evaluating how many calories and fat grams were in the meal I had just eaten.

Added to this was the constant game of comparison that I played out in my mind whenever another woman, particularly an attractive one, walked into the room. *(I'm sorry, did you say something? I was busy guessing your weight.)* This habit became incredibly distracting in public places, such as at the mall or at the office. I would be so focused on how thin everyone else was that I had time for little else.

"Don't Touch My Stomach"

Because we're so convinced that we are grossly fat, many of us recoil from being touched on those parts of ourselves we consider to be the heaviest. For my mother, this was her stomach. She recently told me that during her disorder, she was able to be intimate only if her husband didn't touch her stomach. The very idea of having her stomach touched was—and remains—very uncomfortable to her.

For a friend of mine, this untouchable zone is her thighs. She can feel very attractive with her clothes on, but if her husband touches her thighs, she suddenly feels that they are huge, and she can't stand the reminder that her thighs are, well, there.

"I Must Become Invisible"

For some of us, losing weight means an opportunity to become "invisible" to others, preventing anyone from looking too closely into our lives and discovering that we are not worthy of love and acceptance. When we are thin, we can more easily slip in and out of rooms, virtually unnoticed. I remember that one of my favorite little victories was to be able to slip between chairs that were close together, hoping that someone would notice that I could get through without inconveniencing anyone by making them move. The idea of being small enough to move through life without troubling anyone felt very empowering to me.

My Own Private World

Similar to the empowering feeling of being invisible is the discovery that our dieting makes us feel as if we are in control of something for the first time in our life. Sharon Hersh says, "Eating is one area where we learn early that we can have our own private world."[1] In this place, no one can tell us what to do. No one can control our thoughts. We get to know what is going on while everyone else is in the dark. For those who are living in a very controlled environment, food becomes a way to seek comfort or, conversely, to punish ourselves. Whatever our obsession with eating and weight control entails, we quickly learn that no one can take this private world from us.

"I Must Not Be a Pig"

As a teen I experienced one of the most horrifying and humiliating incidents of my young life while staying with a friend's family for a week or so. I had looked forward to my time there because they had all this great food—Popsicles, chips, and other snacks that we never had at home. I certainly ate my share (and probably more), as any teenager would. Sometime near the end of my visit, my friend's eleven-year-old sister flippantly remarked, "My mom says you're eating us out of house and home." I was horrified. I was ashamed. Keep in mind that this happened a few years before I even had any issues with my weight or with overeating, but the little seed planted by her comment would be sure to raise its ugly head in the years to come. I remember thinking then that I must never again be thought a pig.

I'd like to say that I've never allowed myself to feel this way again, but my most recent experience with this nagging little feeling was not that long ago. I went out to dinner with my girlfriend Jen and another friend. At the time, I was about seven weeks pregnant and suffering from constant and intense nausea. Jen ordered an appetizer—spinach dip—and I found that I couldn't resist having some, hoping that food in my belly would alleviate my nausea. I dug in, really enjoying myself. As I was reaching into the bowl for the fourth or fifth time, Jen put her hand against mine as if to push it away. "You're going to eat all of it," she jokingly said. Wow! A flood of emotions brought me right back to the other times when I had felt humiliated for being a pig. Here I was, having made major progress, having just resigned my job to focus on helping others who struggle in this area, and I was hurt like a baby. I couldn't participate in the rest of the conversation that night. I found myself withdrawing into the safety of my shell. I was humiliated and felt as if I had been chastised.

The following week I came clean with Jen about my feelings. I felt it was important for her to know how fragile some of us can be when it comes to food issues. At the very least, it was a good reminder to me that little seeds planted in us early in life can continue to grow and cause problems later on, even as we make our way toward healing.

"I Can't Miss My Workout"

For many of us, dieting is not enough. Surrounded by images of perfect bodies, we find ourselves wanting more than just to be thin. We argue that if the girl in the commercials can have a completely firm body, then we should be able to achieve one too. If we could just go to the gym every day or run a few miles on a regular basis, then surely our bodies would obey us and look the way we want them to.

As we take steps toward getting into a routine, we gradually become more and more obsessed with the control we feel when we stick with our program. With each minute on the StairMaster, we can literally *feel* the fat coming off, as the handy display screen readily confirms the number of calories being burned. "I just burned off my entire lunch," we think to ourselves, ignoring how light-headed we feel. Proud of our discipline, we walk rubber-legged to the next machine. When we feel too tired to go on, we look around until we find a point of inspiration—someone leaner and more fit than we are. We fixate on her, reasoning that if she can do it, so can we. Before long, our day is strategically planned around our workout, and missing one can compromise our already fragile self-esteem.

There is nothing inherently wrong with working out. When we are in touch with our bodies through physical activity, we benefit mentally, physically, emotionally, and spiritually. What *is* unhealthy, however, is when recreation turns into obsession.

"If I'm Not Thin, They Won't Love Me Anymore"

For most of my life I believed that if I was not thin, I would not be loved. I think some of this came from observing my mother's own frustrating struggles to lose weight. Another factor was that, as I entered my teens, I became more aware of fashion and realized that having a naturally slender figure gave me at least a slight advantage over several other girls my age. This was important to me because during this time I felt very insecure in almost every other area of my life. Being thin became my security blanket.

Throughout the healing process, I've had to learn that a lot of the pressure I felt to be thin was self-imposed, even though I assumed that others expected it of me. Not surprisingly, when I left my position at the record company, I began to experience a greater level of freedom because I was no longer influenced by the perceived expectations of those I had worked so closely with for the previous five years.

So What?

For some reason—each of us has a different one—we've bought into the (false) presumption that people will love us if (and only if) we are thin. Of course, most of us know somewhere in the dusty corners of our brain that this is not true, but it's hard to get that logic from the mind to the soul. Exploring the thought patterns we live with each day helps us determine whether we've crossed the line into an unbalanced view of eating and weight.

Incorporated throughout this book are a series of self-tests and questions, many of which are based on the hard questions I had to ask myself when I first started coming to terms with the way I was living. These exercises are designed to help you evaluate and explore your attitudes and behavior regarding food and dieting.

Read through the following statements and check the ones that are true for you. You might be surprised to realize how many of your thoughts center around food and your weight.

Self-Test No. 1: Thought Processes

- ☑ I keep thinking that if I could just lose a few pounds, everything in life would be better.
- ☐ I feel that a curvy body is not as attractive as one that is bony and thin.
- ☐ I am tired of worrying about weight and food all the time.
- ☐ I am afraid to look in the mirror when I am naked.
- ☑ I frequently look in the mirror to judge my body against the ideal I have in my mind.
- ☐ I pay particular attention to one part of my body. When I notice it getting bigger, I punish myself in some way.
- ☐ A small weight gain can send me into a binge or cause me to significantly limit my eating for several days.
- ☐ Feeling hungry scares me.
- ☐ I have a hard time falling asleep if my belly feels full.

- ☑ I have "fat clothes" for those days when I fear I've gained too much weight.
- ❑ I believe my weight and the size of my body directly affect the respect I get at work and from my peers.
- ☑ I think that people choose whether to accept or reject me based on how I look.
- ❑ Sometimes I wish I could just go someplace totally secluded where I wouldn't have to worry about my weight.

Chapter 4

Weird Eating—Exposed

It is puzzling to me that otherwise sensitive people develop a real docility about the obvious necessity of eating.

—M. F. K. FISHER, culinary writer and autobiographer

The other day I met with a friend who doesn't yet understand that she is a chronic dieter. For some time I have been aware that she often eats unusual things in an effort to stay slim. But when I asked about her eating habits, she told me, "I just make smart choices. If someone gives me a double cheeseburger, I just choose not to eat it." At first this sounded reasonable—until I remembered that it was my own obsession with "smart choices" that eventually led me to a diet consisting of barely enough food to sustain my body.

The unfortunate truth is that too often our desire to lose weight can lead us to a pattern of what I like to call "weird eating"—a dead giveaway that someone has an unhealthy approach to food. Following are some behaviors that indicate when eating has gone beyond choice to obsession.

Dead Giveaways

High-Sugar–Low-Fat Dieting

For many years I maintained a diet that was strictly high sugar–low fat. I felt I needed sugar for energy (plus I was addicted to it), and I avoided fat for obvious reasons. In fact, I was so paranoid of fat that for several years I refused to eat anything that had more than three grams of fat in it, hoping to eat no more than ten grams each day. It took me awhile to learn that including more fat in my diet was not only okay but vital to my health. It is important to note, however, that those who struggle on the bulimic rather than anorexic side of the eating continuum tend toward more fatty foods. As my mother says, "Roast beef and ice cream—the menu of the bulimic." Whatever the specifics of your eating practices, extreme dieting often upsets the normal ratio of calories, fat, and nutrients our bodies need to function well.

Meal Scheduling

Just as we obsess about *what* we can eat, many of us have created very strict rules about *when* we can eat. For example, some of us religiously follow an eating schedule such as 7:00, 12:00, 5:30, regardless of whether we actually feel hungry. Planning our day around mealtimes becomes critical, as we often believe that changing our schedule will have devastating consequences.

Others of us are less concerned about specific times during the day just as long as we don't eat after a certain cutoff point. For example, I used to adamantly insist on eating no later than 6:00 in the evening. I was convinced that if I broke this "rule," the food I ate would not have enough time to metabolize before I went to bed. This was problematic for several reasons. First of all, most of my friends did not live by such strict rules. They would often invite me out to dinner but would want to go at 7:00, 7:30, or even later. In these cases, my only options would be to go and not eat or not to go at all. Another problem was that my work often required me to stay at the office after 6:00 P.M. Because I was dead set against eating any later than that, I would often skip dinner altogether. My unwavering adherence to a strict schedule only made my obsession more difficult to break.

The Nibbler

On the opposite end of the spectrum from the scheduled eater is what I like to call the "nibbler." My friend Danielle is one of these. She won't ever eat a real meal because she is convinced that doing so will make her fat. Instead, she snacks on a lot of little things throughout the day to stave off hunger. Unfortunately, this approach to losing or maintaining weight can actually have the opposite effect, causing increased frustration with eating and even leading to unexpected weight gain.

The first problem with this method is that a nibbler almost never enjoys the satisfaction of eating a real meal. While everyone else is eating a normal-size serving of food, a nibbler tries to convince herself that she's not missing out on anything. Later she may compensate for these feelings of deprivation by binging, which only increases her difficulty in managing her weight.

A second problem is that since a nibbler never eats real meals, her body doesn't know when to anticipate eating, and the normal feelings of hunger and fullness can get mixed up. This, too, can lead to periods of restricting or binging, which often results in further aggravation and weight gain.

A third flaw with this approach to dieting is that often the nibbler ends up eating more throughout the day than if she had just eaten normal meals. By eating such small amounts at a time, nibblers can easily reason away the calories in each nibble, but like it or not, they're still adding up, even if we're not counting. At the end of the day, a nibbler would have been better off simply getting into a routine of eating regular meals.

Ritualistic Behavior

During my college anorexia phase, my eating behaviors became decidedly ritualistic. Not only did I eat only Malt-O-Meal, but I had to cook it in the same pot and eat it with the same spoon every time. As I mentioned earlier, another side to the ritualistic eating patterns of someone who is food obsessed is the extreme aversion to being interrupted during a meal. I would often plan my meals to ensure that no one else was around while I was eating. If someone came into the room, I would either leave or stop eating until the person left. Such an interruption would upset me greatly. I didn't allow myself to eat very often, so when I did, I wanted to be able to focus on every little bite. I wanted to be left alone with my ritual.

"Off-Limits" Foods

Are there foods that you won't touch with a ten-foot pole—and not because you don't like the taste? For many years I would avoid anything that wasn't grilled or steamed, that had cheese or sour cream in it, or that was prepared with milk, butter, or oil, or anything else that represented fat. While this seemed quite acceptable—even reasonable—to me at the time, I have come to realize that I don't need to be so restrictive in order to maintain the normal body type I was born with.

"Safe" Foods

Just as we deem some foods off-limits, we also come up with a list of safe foods. Each list seems to be as different as the individual making it. For me, safe foods were anything without fat. My diet of choice was foods high in carbohydrates—bagels, nonfat candy, cereal (with skim milk), and veggies. Others avoid all carbohydrates, choosing high protein items instead.

The problem with the whole concept of safe foods is that when we consider something to be safe, we often tend to eat more of it. This only perpetuates the binge-starve cycle. And from a health standpoint, by limiting our diet to a smaller variety of foods, we can be missing out on nutrients that are essential to our overall health.

Nutrition Information Label Fixation

Fixating on the numbers listed on nutrition information labels has become a necessary part of life for most chronic dieters. With most food products clearly displaying the FDA-required labels, it has become easier to accept or reject certain foods in our diet.

For some of us, calories are the biggest factor, and we carefully calculate every meal so as not to exceed a certain total for the day. Others are more concerned about fat grams, convinced that if they can just keep their total fat intake low enough, they will lose weight. With the popularity of diets such as the Dr. Atkins method of weight loss, many dieters focus instead on the total number of carbohydrates they consume. And while there are an increasing number of arguments to suggest that limiting our carbohydrate intake can actually be a positive move, plans like Dr. Atkins's require a constant and obsessive attention to even the tiniest traces of caloric value.

For example, one low-carb newsgroup offers a warning about foods such as cream, eggs, and sugar-free gum that contain "hidden carbs," although each of these actually has less than one gram of carbohydrate per serving. By placing an emphasis on such small quantities of a food group, dieters open themselves up to an increased anxiety about everything they eat. Consider this posting I found on the same newsgroup Web site: "I must not carb. Carbs are the diet-killer. Carbs are the little-binge that will bring total obliteration...."

The intensity of this posting reflects the obsessive nature of those of us who become almost fanatical in our weight-control efforts. Once we come up with a plan that we think will work for us, we become consumed with the details of carrying out that plan, right down to the last gram.

Fad Diets

Like the example above, many fad diets encourage weird eating in an effort to trick the body into losing weight. Sometimes this can mean eliminating certain foods, or even entire food groups, from one's diet. At other times, it means adopting an unusual pattern of eating, as with programs that require strict adherence to a certain diet for six days followed by a free day on the seventh. One of my friends is currently on a plan like this and has lost quite a bit of weight...but it hasn't come without a price. When I asked her how the program was working for her, she admitted that the temptation to binge on the free day was overwhelming. Just the week before, she had really pigged out. "I felt so bad I wanted to throw up," she told me. I found this to be somewhat alarming, as purging was not something she had ever considered before going on the diet.

The truth is, while fad diets may indeed produce the desired results for a time, once dieters achieve their weight-loss goal, their only option for maintenance is to continue a pattern of weird eating. This causes many problems, from frustration-induced binge eating to a fixation on off-limits and safe foods to certain health implications that are unique to each dieter. Because of these and other factors, fad diets often cause more harm than good.

Fasting

"I am doing really good.... I have been fasting for twenty-five days, and I actually allowed myself a Diet Coke today, so I guess that's a good thing," writes Aly on a proanorexia ("pro-ana") Web site. While Aly's comment may sound extreme to some people, fasting has become a popular weight-loss method for women and men of all ages and sizes.

In ancient times, fasting was often undertaken as a means by which to seek and honor God. In the church today, fasting is still regarded as a sign of spirituality and the ultimate act of denial for the purpose of hearing from God. Even for those outside religious circles, fasting is often seen as a socially acceptable way to exert perfect control over one of the most difficult things to tame: our appetite.

Unfortunately, fasting often leads to disordered eating, even for those who aren't weight obsessed to begin with. It is also a terrible weight-control method. For one thing, during a fast our body enters into a state of starvation, during which it tries to compensate for the lack of food by holding on to whatever fat stores we have available.

As we continue to fast, our brain loses its ability to manufacture the calming agent serotonin, and we can find ourselves obsessing about food and our weight. During this time, our views about our body can become even more distorted than they already were. At the beginning of our fast, we might have wanted to lose a few pounds, but by the end of it, we may feel even fatter than when we began—even if we've lost weight.

Once the fast is over, we are faced with an impossible choice: continue to starve or risk gaining back all of the weight we've lost. The stress caused by this dilemma can trigger binge eating and yo-yo dieting, which is why so many people who fast regain all the weight they lost, and often more.

Because of realities like these, fasting is an unrealistic and even dangerous means of weight control. And while I can appreciate the role of fasting for spiritual or medical reasons, I strongly discourage the practice for anyone who is prone to obsessing about food and weight.

Organic Obsessions and Orthorexia

Many well-intentioned healthy eaters unknowingly enter into yet another type of disordered behavior when they become obsessed with eating only pure, raw, or organic foods. After struggling for years as a self-described "extreme eater," Dr. Steven Bratman coined the term *orthorexia* to describe an obsession with so-called healthy eating.[1] The ANRED Web site states, "Orthorexics obsess over what to eat, how much to eat, how to prepare food 'properly,' and where to obtain 'pure' and 'proper' foods." They also "feel superior to others who eat 'improper' foods, which might include non-organic or junk foods and items found in regular grocery stores, as opposed to health food stores."[2] Again, at issue here is the loss of balance. By placing such a heightened importance on every ingredient of the food that is eaten, the orthorexic is no better off than the anorexic, bulimic, or binge eater when it comes to the hold that food and eating have on their lives.

Binge-Starve Cycles

It seems that most of us who obsess about food and our weight have struggled, or still struggle, with a binge-starve eating pattern. I am referring to the times when we decide we deserve a normal meal. Then we feel a little guilty for eating, so we decide to "make it better" by eating more. Before we know it, we've totally pigged out, and now we feel really gross. So we decide we're going to starve the next day to make up for it. The problem with the binge-starve cycle is that it often becomes a repeated pattern that we can't seem to shake.

Caffeine

While an addiction to caffeine isn't always related to disordered eating, many of us who diet are drawn to highly caffeinated drinks to boost our otherwise non-existent energy level and to keep ourselves from feeling hungry.

I remember a time when I drank at least a twelve-pack of Diet Coke each day. When I got too cold, I switched to drinking coffee with little or no cream. Whatever it took, I kept the caffeine flowing. Eventually, my habit gave me the jitters and disrupted my sleep patterns to the point that I had to drink more caffeine just to fall asleep. I've since sworn off caffeine altogether and am much better off.

Pills, Supplements, and Teas

I doubt that any of us have seen a supplement that actually has long-term weight-loss benefits for ourselves or others we know. Many people continue to abuse supplements, however, in hopes of finding a perfect method for their weight-loss madness. One of my friends told me in tears one night that she had seen a certain supplement working wonders with another girl we both knew, and she was desperate to try it but couldn't afford the relatively high price tag. She felt that if she could just take this pill, her problems with weight would be solved.

Another friend admitted to me that for several years she had been drinking a supplemental tea that contained ephedrine to increase her energy so that she could dedicate more time to maintaining her weight and exercising. Five years after she first started drinking the tea, she began to experience serious health problems that were attributable to the ingredients of the tea. Even so, while she knew she should throw it away, she held on to the tea in much the same way a smoker holds on to her last pack…just in case.

Whatever your diet accelerator of choice, the important thing to remember is that nothing apart from a consistent eating pattern is ever going to help you achieve a healthy body weight.

You will throw away thousands of dollars just to back-pedal in your own progress unless you make an earnest decision to come to terms with your situation and seek out help along the way.

Colonics and Cleanses

For many of us, our obsession with dieting extends to ensuring that we *eliminate* the food we eat before it can make us gain weight. Sometimes these efforts can be decidedly weird.

In September 2002 VH1 and *Self* magazine partnered to produce *Rock Bodies,* a televised report that explored the truth behind how certain celebrities get and maintain their "perfect" bodies. The report showed that many people, including celebrities, have turned to colonics to help rid them of unwanted weight.

In case you're wondering if a colonic is as bad as it sounds, rest assured—it is. The procedure entails shooting a stream of purified water up into the colon (ouch!). As the water goes in, the toxins come out. Beginning at around one hundred dollars a pop, this treatment can become an expensive, not to mention uncomfortable, method for weight loss. And while most people who have colonics do experience some weight loss, it is not without its downsides.

Joy Bauer, a nutrition expert interviewed for *Rock Bodies,* says, "Colonics don't make you skinny, [they] dehydrate you. You feel thinner for the moment because you lose some water weight, but as soon as you eat or drink, the weight is back on."[3] Dr. Steven Lamm of NYU Medical Center adds, "A three-week program of fasting and colonics is potentially dangerous. You can induce electrolyte imbalance and potassium deficiency."[4]

Those of us who don't have the tolerance (or the cash) for such an intrusive procedure may experiment with supplemental cleanses. Normally combined with some sort of fasting, cleanses involve taking pills that are designed to rid the body of toxins. I once tried one of these cleanses to lose weight, and it worked— I couldn't leave the bathroom for days. I ended up stopping before the program was complete, deciding that anything was better than relentless diarrhea.

The truth we need to understand is that all of our weird efforts to control our diets and our bodies only make us more frustrated and push us further into our obsessive behaviors.

So What?

As with our thought processes, our weird eating habits can become so much a part of our lives that we don't even notice them. We ignore the importance of a balanced diet and tell ourselves that others aren't aware of our strange behaviors. But even if no one else knows the lengths to which we are willing to go, weird eating and food obsession will definitely take their toll.

Self-Test No. 2: Weird Eating

❑ Instead of eating a "real" meal, I frequently eat empty calories such as candy or chips (especially if they're fat free).

❑ When I'm eating out, I always ask for foods to be specially prepared (without butter, oils, or cheese, etc.).

❑ A typical lunch for me is Diet Coke or coffee and fruit or a dinner salad (for example: just greens—no meat, no cheese, no extras).

❑ I won't eat anything if I don't know how many calories and/or fat grams are in it.

❑ I frequently make a meal out of low-fat microwave popcorn.

❑ I won't eat a slice of pizza, but I'll eat everyone's leftover crusts.

❑ I've learned how to look as if I'm eating a lot even when I'm not.

❑ My friends tell me my eating habits are weird.

❑ If I eat (what I consider to be) too much at lunch, then I'll probably skip dinner.

❑ If I eat (what I consider to be) too much one day, then I'll probably try not to eat the next day.

❑ Sometimes I skip out on social functions because I don't want to have to eat what is being served.

❑ Even though I don't let myself eat what I want to, I actually love to eat.

❑ My weight would not be considered too thin by today's standards (on television).

❑ My goal is to eat less than 1,500 calories a day.

❑ A good day is when I don't eat anything on my "restricted" list.

❑ I am tired of thinking about eating (and being thin) all the time.

Health and Physiological Factors

Our bodies are able to tolerate enormous amounts of abuse, but sooner or
later they begin to break down.

—GREGORY L. JANTZ, PH.D., *Hope, Help, and Healing for Eating Disorders*

Weird eating has its price. Depending on our type of dieting and weight
control, we may begin to see a number of physical symptoms manifest
themselves. These symptoms, if left unchecked, can cause significant problems
later in life. Symptoms include:

- headaches
- dizziness
- insomnia
- heart palpitations
- shortness of breath
- irregular menstrual cycles
- skin pallor
- chronic halitosis (bad breath)
- frequent or chronic fatigue
- stomach cramps
- weakness
- constant hunger
- tooth enamel loss
- irritability
- mood swings
- loss of sexual interest

- yeast infections
- depressed mood
- dysentery
- infrequent bowel movements/constipation
- osteoporosis (early onset)
- body aches

You may be surprised to see some of these symptoms on the list. Many people associate physical changes such as these with more extreme eating disorders. For instance, you may know that bulimics suffer from the erosion of tooth enamel as a result of their constant purging. I was surprised to learn that chronic dieters can suffer similar problems since the high level of acid generated in the stomachs of those who don't eat enough can still make its way to their mouth. A person with EDNOS may not experience the same extreme physical symptoms as someone with full-blown anorexia or bulimia, but treating your body unnaturally will eventually result in some physical distress.

Personality Changes

People who are healthy and maintain a balanced diet seem to have a more steady personality than those who struggle in the area of eating. Many of us with disordered eating suffer not only physiologically but also mentally, emotionally, and spiritually, which can have a significant impact on our temperament.

Social Dysfunction and Withdrawal

My social activity was very sporadic during my years of disordered eating. Sometimes I would feel energized and become the proverbial social butterfly, commanding attention in social settings. At other times, I would be entirely caught up in thinking about what food was being served. During the binge phases of my disorder, I would be completely unaware of anything going on in the room other than how much food I could eat. And in the starve phases, I would avoid certain social situations altogether to keep from being tempted by any bad foods that I might not be able to resist. I remember one such occasion when our church was having a spaghetti dinner after the morning service. I badly wanted to go, as my husband and I had not yet had the opportunity to interact socially with many of the members. However, the day before had been a bad eating day for me, and I felt I couldn't be around food at all. So we missed out on this social opportunity—and many others—because of my obsessive fear.

Contributing to my social struggles was the fact that, like many disordered eaters (particularly those who diet excessively), I often felt scattered in social settings. One reason for this is the internal war raging in our minds. We're so busy comparing, obsessing, and worrying that it's difficult to carry on a fluid conversation. Another reason is the fact that our undernourished brain sometimes has a difficult time processing normally, causing us to lose our train of thought or to feel sort of spaced out. Our insecurity may also prevent us from truly engaging with others. We often put up a sort of shield, afraid to let anyone get too close for fear they'll see us for the pitiful souls we feel we are.

Mood Swings

I have experienced many intensely crippling mood swings during my years of unhealthy eating. Again, this often comes down to a physiological issue. The brain is not getting all the nourishment it requires, and in return, our emotional nerve centers are affected.

When I was pregnant, however, I was startled one day to realize that it had been quite some time since I had experienced a noticeable mood swing. It was during this period of more normal eating habits that I found I had a much more even-tempered personality. While some of this may have been due to the fact that I was living a much less stressful life than I did when I worked full time, I attribute most of it to the fact that my body and brain were getting more of what they needed to function properly. Even after the pregnancy, when many women suffer through incredibly intense mood swings as a result of drastically changing hormones, I seemed to keep an even keel. This has made my life (and my husband's) so much easier.

"I Don't Need Anyone"

I don't completely understand it, but there is something about succumbing to this disorder that makes many of us feel this strange independence, where we push others away while at the same time longing desperately for friendship and interaction. It is a strange dichotomy that I've experienced on several levels. During my anorexic phase I began to notice that I was withdrawing from my roommates and friends. Not long after that I realized I had an extreme aversion to even catching the eye of one of my classmates in the hallway. I withdrew further and further into this shell, all the while proud of myself for doing quite well on the whole losing weight thing. It was during this period that my thought life became the most self-destructive. Even as I worked to avoid personal contact with most everyone, I was becoming lonelier and lonelier, to the point of despair.

Consider this journal entry, written that year:

> My relationships are falling apart.
> I hate living with my roommates.
> My classes are going in one ear and out the other.
> Most times I don't even want to be here.
> I have to consciously force myself to be nice to others.
> I am not sensitive to others like I have been in the past.
> I make no effort to share anything.
> I prance around every day as if I'm God's gift to creation, yet I don't feel
>   that anyone wants me around. So I've just decided not to care—I
>   don't need them anyway.
> I'm lonely!
> I seem to burn my bridges behind me. One major cause is fear of
>   rejection—"Surely they don't want me around anymore."
> I run away from people. I never walk to or from school with anyone. I
>   am always by myself.
> I am an island.

I can easily remember the pain and rejection that I felt, which was, oddly enough, the result of my own actions.

A few years later, as I settled into a pattern of chronic dieting, I experienced a different side of this problem. Even as I found myself pursued by men and surrounded by a wonderful new circle of friends, I couldn't seem to trust anyone to get close to me. I soon realized that I was running on empty. Not only was I hungry for food, I was emotionally barren. I could flare up at the simplest thing.

Intolerance Toward People Because of Their Size

In the midst of disordered eating, we can find it difficult to realize that others are struggling with the same demons we do. We see someone who appears to be thinner than we are, and we hate that person because of her size. Or we might have an unhealthy and even arrogant intolerance of those who struggle with being overweight.

Because we've placed such an intense focus on being thin and in control, we find it hard to respect anyone who falls short of the standards we esteem so highly. Of course, this only exacerbates the problem when we ourselves put on weight or have a hard time getting thin. With a sense of horror, we imagine ourselves being associated with those we've openly criticized, and we fearfully decide that our only option is to get our act together and our weight under control.

The important point here is that the further we move into our disordered eating behavior, the less we are able to allow for different standards when it comes to weight, whether for ourselves or for those around us.

So What?

Subclinical eating disorders may not have the same extreme symptoms of clinical disorders, which is part of the reason they are so dangerous. When we eliminate specific foods and/or entire food groups through weird eating or excessive dieting, we are choosing to deprive our bodies of the nutrients and other healthful substances they need to function well. And while to some of us this may seem a risk worth taking, it is only a matter of time before our bodies will begin to evidence signs of breakdown.

Self-Test No. 3: Health and Physiological Indicators

1. Check any symptom you live with daily:
   - ❑ headaches
   - ❑ dizziness
   - ❑ insomnia
   - ❑ heart palpitations
   - ❑ shortness of breath
   - ❑ irregular menstrual cycles
   - ❑ skin pallor
   - ❑ chronic halitosis (bad breath)
   - ❑ frequent or chronic fatigue
   - ❑ stomach cramps
   - ❑ weakness
   - ❑ constant hunger
   - ❑ irritability
   - ❑ mood swings
   - ❑ lack of sexual interest
   - ❑ yeast infections
   - ❑ depressed mood
   - ❑ dysentery
   - ❑ infrequent bowel movements/constipation
   - ❑ osteoporosis (early onset)
   - ❑ body aches

2. In what ways have you noticed your personality changing since you've become more concerned with dieting (i.e., mood swings that make you irritable, intolerance of others)?

3. Do your symptoms seem significant enough for you to consider changing the way you eat? Why or why not?

Prayer

God, help me to be willing to explore whether my attitudes toward eating and weight control are healthy and balanced.

Give me wisdom to see which things I've come to believe about myself and my body are untrue.

Help me walk forward in this process of self-discovery; shine a light on each next step I should take.

I want to walk in truth.

PART 2

HOW DID WE GET HERE?

As we become more aware of our unhealthy views on eating and weight, it's natural to think, *I never wanted to be here. How did I get here?*

As I began asking myself this question, I found it helpful to understand that many factors contributed to my problem. Being able to look back and recognize those things that served as catalysts along the way helped me begin unraveling the web of lies I had come to believe about myself and my body.

In this section, we'll explore several of the factors that contribute to disordered eating. The questions that appear at the end of each chapter are designed to help you in your own process of self-discovery. Because all of us struggle in different ways, you may find that some chapters really speak to you, while others don't seem to apply. So as you read, feel free to move ahead to those chapters that speak to you more personally.

This is a personal journey for each of us.

Chapter 6

We Live in a
Fallen World

Psychology keeps trying to vindicate human nature. History keeps undermining the effort.

—MASON COOLEY, *City Aphorisms, Fifth Selection*

When considering how we came to believe that being thin was worth pursuing at any cost, we must start by examining more closely the flaws of our humanity. Regardless of our own personal belief systems, we probably all agree that the world we live in is far from perfect. Watching just a ten-minute segment of the evening news will back this up, as we are inundated with images of murder, rape, theft, school shootings, and war. We have only to flip a channel to become overwhelmed with messages touting the importance of success, beauty, achievement, and sex appeal. There is little that is inherently redeeming about this world.

Genesis tells the story of the very beginning of the human race and of a choice to eat forbidden fruit that resulted in broken fellowship with God. Since that momentous decision, our world has never again been the same. In its well-read pages, the Bible details countless stories of war, murder, conflict, and persecution, all of which followed what regrettably was a very short time in Eden. And so we live in a fallen world. By the simple fact of our humanity, we are all predisposed to sin and weakness in this life on earth. It's important to understand how this predisposition has shaped us.

Our Human Nature

The other day my neighbor, a marketing professional specializing in direct-mail advertising, told me that in order for an advertisement to be successful, its message must speak to one of the following: greed, fear, or sex. *An interesting commentary on our culture at large,* I thought. As I considered this further, I realized that these elements of our human nature can explain the driving force behind nearly every type of problem we struggle with.

Greed

This sixteenth-century word, defined by *Webster's Dictionary* as "excessive or reprehensible acquisitiveness," actually originates from the word *greedy,* which appeared two centuries earlier. Interestingly, the first definition for *greedy* is "having a strong desire for food or drink." This is easier to appreciate when we consider that in earlier centuries money, fame, and possessions were not pursued the way they are today, which made eating and drinking two of the most indulgent activities.

Although greed looks a bit different today, our society remains consumed with the pursuit of having more. Our yearning for importance is insatiable. We hungrily desire success. To gain these things, we believe that we must be beautiful, and to be beautiful, we must be thin. After all, as the saying goes, "You can never be too rich or too thin."

But the same forces that drive us to be thin also tell us we can have it all. Ads for food often feature thin and gorgeous models, implying that we can eat our cake and still have a perfect body. So we greedily assemble our arsenal of weight-reduction methods. No cost is too great in our effort to attain the thinness that represents our value. And, as is true in cases of greed, the more we get (or lose, in the case of weight), the more we want.

Yes, greed is a force to be reckoned with when it comes to finding balance in our lives.

Fear

No matter how many good things are happening in our lives, we are often dominated by fear. We fear the loss of our job because that would jeopardize our finances, self-worth, and future. We fear the discovery that we are not healthy because that would mean our lives might not end up the way we have planned, and the idea of becoming a burden to others is almost more than we can bear. We fear being taken advantage of. We fear losing the respect of others. We fear not finding a mate and never having the chance to have children of our own.

Is it any surprise, then, that fear is quite often our strongest motivator for pursuing thinness? In our minds, fat equals unlovable, undesirable, unsuccessful, unworthy, unattractive, unhealthy, and a myriad of other "un's" that we could add to the list. So it is only logical that we have come to believe that being thin will enable us to overcome our fears. We think, *If I'm thin, they'll value me more at my job, and I'll never have to worry about getting laid off.* Or, *If only I could lose weight, then I would have so many more friends and would never feel alone.* Similarly, when it comes to actually choosing to accept our natural weight, the fear of what others think can seem like a formidable roadblock. The important thing to realize is that fear, while definitely a strong motivator, rarely motivates us positively.

Sex Appeal

As humans, our most basic physical desire after water and food (though some would reverse that order) is sex. But while sex is a God-given pleasure and an important part of our humanity, we often place undue focus on attaining the perfect sexy body. Should we have any doubts as to what that means, the media continually reminds us that a flat stomach and thin thighs are much more desirable than an hourglass figure. (Strange, considering that two of the defining characteristics of a woman are her softness and curves.)

Talk shows often glorify the pursuit of such standards of thinness, taking delight in bringing onstage the high-school crushes of formerly heavy girls who now flaunt their newly sculpted bodies as if to say, "See what you're missing now?" Supportively, we cheer them on, proud of their efforts to conform to our culture's rigid standards of what is sexy. Once in a while someone speaks up and says, "But you don't have any breasts now," but no one pays attention. Perhaps that seems a small price to pay for the admiring glances these women have acquired as a result of their efforts. But to the observant viewer, it is apparent that for all their newfound power, these women literally tremble with insecurity, their body language belying a screaming need for true acceptance. Even in their moment of glory, these women are no closer to accepting themselves than when they took up a whole seat on the school bus.

When we are ruled by a desire to be sexy, we become willing participants in defeating our "self" in the pursuit of a body that has been modeled to us by the media. Too often we forget that those who are modeling such standards are usually trapped in their own thin cage.

The Porn Parallel

Recently I was traveling to a conference as the guest of a friend. Riding on the bus with her band, I fell into a conversation with one of her musicians about the quest for perfection that often leads to eating disorders and image issues. As we talked, Michael startled me with a stunning comparison that I had never considered. "You know," he said, "I would imagine that the hold that eating and image issues have on women can only be compared to the hold that pornography often has on us guys." What an amazing statement! Since that discussion, nearly every man I have talked with about this subject understands it better when I mention this parallel.

Consider that an addiction to pornography often starts small, with an adult magazine or a risqué movie. With that first small taste, the viewer is hooked. The next time it takes a little more to satisfy the longing. This is where more addictive behaviors can come in, the person becomes more deviant and deceptive, the images of sexual escapades playing out in his mind with increased frequency. Because of the stigma associated with such behavior, the person is often compelled to start living a secret life, stealing time away from relationships to feed his ever-increasing appetite for sexual satisfaction.

If you've struggled at all with disordered eating and chronic dieting, you know that the pattern is eerily similar. In the beginning it starts with just a little idea of what it would mean to be thin, to achieve the perfect body. Next, as we start to "give a little ground" (as my dad would say), we begin to find ourselves sucked in by the aphrodisiac of power and control. The further we get into it, the more obsessed we become, until our every thought is consumed with food and weight: *What will I eat? Am I thin enough? I'm not thin enough. Oh, no. I ate too much. My stomach's too big. These pants feel tighter than they did the last time I wore them. I'm such a gross, fat pig,* and so on. But in spite of the frustrating dominance of these thoughts, we are too embarrassed to admit our struggle, leaving many of our friends and loved ones completely unaware that we have a problem at all.

And while these similarities are striking, another factor makes the comparison even more powerful: The illusion of total control. Leanne Spencer explains,

> The person who struggles with pornography thinks, *When I am alone with a pornographic magazine or Internet site or am watching an adult video, I am in control of everything I am feeling. I do not have to enter into a deep relationship with the other person. I do not have obligations to her. I decide when and where it happens and how often. I take what is actually my inability to feel safe with another human and control it all for myself so that I feel safe. I am the captain of my ship.*
>
> Similarly, the disordered eater thinks, *This is a game I play by myself. I decide what I eat, what foods are safe or not safe, and what new technique I will use to control my weight. Instead of entering a deep, nurturing relationship with others, I keep my true self at a distance. I make my body an object I can manipulate because it is through that control that I am able to feel safe. In my little world I can play all the games I want—I deny food and feel the rush; I eat too much and feel the condemnation. The goal is to spend time being in control so that I can feel "good" and "safe" and "satisfied."*[1]

Of course, not all who struggle with pornography are men, and likewise, disordered eating can affect both men and women. But it's interesting to see the parallels between these two types of addiction. Both require secrecy; both require control; both dictate that the person decide how he or she will be satisfied. And both are seemingly obvious traps, yet so many fall into them.

The Cult of Thin?

In ancient times, people worshiped idols of all sorts in hopes that they might be blessed with fertility, rain, healthy livestock, and fruitful harvests. For many of us today, our body has become our god. If not our only god, it certainly is an object of worship to us. Daily we give of our time, money, and energy to pay homage to her. Hoping to receive her blessing (thinness), we gladly offer sacrifices, such as spending an extra thirty minutes on the StairMaster or refusing dessert. We adorn her with makeup and trendy clothing so that others will see that she is worthy of their worship too.

In her provocative book *Am I Thin Enough Yet? The Cult of Thinness and the Commercialization of Identity*, Sharlene Hesse-Biber explores the ways in which our culture has deified having a thin body. As she notes the sacrifices so many of us are willing to make to be thin, she draws a strong comparison between those who are weight obsessed and members of religious cults. She writes,

> In both cases a group of individuals is committed to a life defined by a rigid set of values and rules. Members of true cults frequently isolate themselves from the rest of the world and develop a strong sense of community. They seem obsessed with the path to perfection, which, though unattainable, holds out compelling promises. In following their ideals, they usually feel that they are among "the chosen."[2]

When I read this I was blown away. Hesse-Biber was describing me and nearly every other person I know who struggles with weight obsession. I had never thought of my behavior as being cultlike before, but when I was presented with these and other similarities, it was hard to avoid the truth. I can easily remember how methodical and rigid I was when it came to counting calories and avoiding certain foods, intent on keeping my "god" happy. And when my efforts paid off, I honestly thought myself to be more enlightened than those who couldn't seem to lose weight.

It's not hard to find people who have very specific rules for how they live, all in the name of controlling their weight. For instance, I recently came across a revealing poem posted on a Web site devoted to those pursuing a low-carb lifestyle. Following is a short segment:

The "Order" of Atkins
We take communion with WASA crackers
We eat the flesh of dead animals!
We chant…ketosis…ketosis…ketosis…[3]

While I can appreciate the intended levity in this poem (it was posted in a section called "Low-Carb Humor"), I've been around enough low-carb dieters to know that these words accurately reflect the kinds of thoughts many of them live with daily. And while they may not realize how rigid their lifestyle has become, their fervor echoes the cultlike mentality to which Hesse-Biber refers.

The fact is, regardless of our size or our method of dieting, anyone whose life becomes ruled by the dos and don'ts of weight loss has unknowingly entered the so-called cult of thinness.

So What?

In order to effectively break free from our obsession with weight, we must first understand that, because we are human, we are often going to be inclined to do what might not be healthy for us.

1. How do greed, fear, and sex appeal play into your obsession with being thin?

2. Do you think your body has become a god in your life? What are some specific ways you worship it?

3. Do you see any similarities between your lifestyle and living within the confines of a cult? Explain.

Chapter 7

How Our Past Shaped Us

The beginning sets the rules.

—MASON COOLEY, *City Aphorisms, Eleventh Selection*

There is no escaping the fact that certain events and circumstances in our past have shaped us in seemingly unalterable ways. Of course, there's been no small amount of discussion over the years about repressed memories and childhood traumas, and such extensive focus on these issues has caused many of us to shrug them off as just another excuse for unhealthy and destructive behaviors. But I think it's important to allow ourselves to go back in time and evaluate which things—positive and negative—helped fashion our sense of self.

The Family Factor

I have the utmost respect and love for my parents. Through the toughest of circumstances, including their divorce, they did everything they could to provide a loving home for us. My father, an incredibly hard-working man, taught me the value of being responsible and doing my part, even when it meant rolling up my sleeves and getting dirty. He remains an ever-present voice of wisdom in my life, a touchstone I still depend on in times of decision.

My mother, a sensitive woman with an interest in the arts, continually encouraged us to discover and share our talents. A "gifter" by nature, she also taught me the importance of thoughtful and unexpected acts of kindness toward others. I have many fond memories of our special one-on-one times together.

Both of my parents have sacrificed much for me, my older sister, and my younger brother, so it is with great care and respect that I tread into the long-stilled waters of the past.

Attitudes About Weight

Having struggled with her weight since childhood, my mother had her first "success" with weight loss around the time I was born. "I was chronically dieting while I was pregnant with you," she recently told me. "No one told me I shouldn't, so by the time you were born, I had actually lost eleven pounds during the pregnancy. Back then I didn't realize that there were books that listed the calories in foods. It wasn't until later that I realized I was eating only five hundred to seven hundred calories a day! But at the time I had no idea I was being unhealthy. I thought I was just doing the right thing by finally staying on a diet."

As I was growing up, my mother's struggles with weight and dieting were always present in our home. A picture she had hung on our refrigerator depicted a model who apparently represented the target weight Mom was shooting for. Mom started going to Weight Watchers and even became a lecturer for them, all the while still struggling to accept her own weight. At times Mom would be on a specific diet and would eat differently from the rest of us. She would also overeat quite frequently, which only served to increase her frustration.

My father had a difficult time with Mom's weight. As younger children, my siblings and I were not aware of this, but as we grew older, it was generally understood in our family that it was undesirable to be overweight.

When I was about nine, my mother again fell into a struggle with disordered eating, but this time our lives became more directly affected by her problem. Now my siblings and I were old enough to observe what was happening. As Mom exhibited strange and unusual eating patterns, each of us undoubtedly took away something different from the experience. Despite all that was happening in our home, I never felt as though either parent thought my siblings or I needed to lose weight. I believe, however, that the ever-present obsessive attitude about weight in my childhood home served as a catalyst that caused me to freak out when I first put on those extra pounds in college.

Forbidden Foods

Because my mother struggled so much with her weight, she was afraid for her children and was determined to make sure that we would not suffer the same way she had as a child. Her response to this understandable fear was to keep us away from foods that most children are allowed to have. On the "forbidden" list were candy bars, cookies, ice cream, chocolate, and other childhood favorites. While we were occasionally allowed to have such foods, we definitely got the message that, for the most part, they were off-limits.

What made these strict limits more difficult was the fact that Mom was always involved in some sort of food-oriented activity such as cake decorating or chocolate making. (Frequent cooking and baking are common practices for those with disordered eating.) We would smell the cakes baking and see all the wonderful sweets, but we were not allowed to partake of them. Never one to leave things to chance, Mom even put a note in the sugar bowl that read, "Please do not eat the sugar—God is watching."

Recently my mom and I talked about these rules, and she could hardly believe what she had done so many years ago. For all her faulty methods, her intentions were pure: She was simply trying to prevent us from having to struggle with weight as she had. The unfortunate side to this was that I soon began to place an unhealthy importance on eating sweet and sugary foods—a sort of rebellion against the rules at home.

It is human nature to seek what is most unattainable. So when I left the confines of my home and went out to fend for myself at college, the first thing I did was run to all the forbidden foods I had longed for as a child. I think that if I had been allowed to incorporate these foods into a regular diet while I was growing up, I would not have binged on them the first chance I got. This is not to say that we should bring our children up to eat sweets all the time. I do think it's important, however, that we choose wisely which items we prohibit them from enjoying. Often, the very items we forbid or limit will be built up in the mind of a child and become far more important than they should be.

Food as Reward and Punishment

It is common in our culture to use food as a reward—I find myself doing this with my own son. A classic example of this is the promise, "Be good in the store, and Mommy will give you a treat." Indeed, food and the activity of eating were intended to be pleasurable. But it's important not to *overemphasize* the role of food as a reward, since this can send the message that eating is more than a normal and enjoyable part of our everyday lives. The child who is *always* rewarded with food grows into the adult who reasons away her overeating, saying, "I *deserve* this carton of ice cream. I've earned it!"

Adding to our confusion about the proper role of food is its use as a form of punishment. For example, when I was a child, my parents experimented with making us miss dinner as a consequence for wrongdoing. While many parents consider this an effective punishment, I personally think it is not a healthy one.

Using food as a punishment or a reward communicates that food and bad or good behavior are linked. It is only logical that these mixed messages can cause problems later in life when we turn to food for comfort or abstain from food as penance.

Longing for Approval

A key factor in my struggles with self-acceptance was a constant and unmet desire for praise from my father. This was a difficult area for him because he had been raised to believe that pride was a thing to be avoided at any cost. So he held back from praising us kids out of concern that we would become prideful. As a result, I grew up feeling the need to do more, to be more, just so that Dad would be pleased with me—and show it.

As I grew older, I felt my figure was something that would surely gain me Dad's praise. Since I knew him to be weight conscious, staying thin seemed a logical way to guarantee his approval. It was this assumption that caused me to worry when I first put on weight at college. I was sure that Dad would think I was fat. The interesting thing is that even at my heaviest, my father thought I looked fine. It turns out that our standards of thin were dramatically different.

Looking back, I can see how my constant, unfulfilled pursuit of my father's approval grew into an unquenchable thirst for approval from nearly everyone I came into contact with. As I walked through this discovery process with my counselor, I had the opportunity to talk with Dad about these issues and was able to finally make peace with them. Now my father seems to take a special interest in me and in the things I'm doing. I no longer feel the need to fight so hard for his approval.

Trouble in the Schoolyard

For most of us growing up in the public or private school system, each day brought about new pressures to fit in. We learned that unless we were cute, wore the latest styles, were good at sports, or were friends with the right people, we were worthless. Day after day we endured the "arrows" that often plunge in deepest when they're shot from the bow of our peers. One sure bet was that the "fat girl" always got picked on. For most of us, that was reason enough to make sure we never found ourselves in that position.

Less obvious perhaps than the teasing was the constant underlying message, "You must fit in to be loved." Fitting in is difficult for any child. The beauty of becoming an adult is that we have the luxury of selecting our own social environment, which makes fitting in an easier task. But when we were children, choosing our environment was not an option, so we learned at an early age to do whatever it took to make sure we weren't the ones who were jeered at, picked on, and scorned.

Today things are exponentially worse for young children. According to some studies, 81 percent of ten-year-olds are afraid of being fat.[1] Forty-two percent of first- through third-grade girls want to be thinner, and more than half of nine- and ten-year-old girls say they feel better about themselves if they are on a diet.[2] The situation has grown so extreme, Hesse-Biber writes, that "self-imposed malnutrition has become a health concern in clinical pediatric practice."[3]

Although we can't get our own childhood back, it is important that we do everything we can to support and encourage the children around us. Scars from one's youth often go deep, and they rarely heal completely. As children head into adolescence, a positive self-image can mean the difference between self-acceptance and self-punishment.

Trauma and Abuse

Quite often some type of trauma or abuse—whether experienced as a child or an adult or both—has played a part in our obsession with being thin. Following are just a few of the factors that can feed this obsession.

Traumatic Events

For many of us who have been victims of divorce, the trauma associated with the breakdown of our family unit can be profound. During such times some people turn to food to ease the pain and rejection they feel. Others may retreat into the "safety" of a restricted diet to prove to themselves that not everything in their lives is falling apart.

Trauma less obvious than divorce can have equally distressing effects, particularly when we are young. For example, one nine-year-old girl tells the story of a day in gym class when all the girls surrounded her and started poking her stomach and calling her fat. Following this traumatic event, the broken and humiliated girl tried vomiting for the first time.[4]

Sexual Abuse

Disordered eating can also be common among people who have been molested or are involved in a sexually abusive relationship. For those who feel they've been trespassed against, exerting strict control over what they eat can be a way to reclaim their right to their own bodies. Others who are abused sexually might turn to food for comfort and then grow fearful when even the size of their body seems to be out of their control. And because the healthy role of sex is compromised in cases of sexual abuse, a heightened sense of the importance of being sexy and attractive can make an already complicated situation worse.

Mental and Emotional Abuse

While traumatic events and sexual abuse can be easy to recognize, any time imbalance occurs in our relationships, there is opportunity for abuse, whether mental, emotional, physical, or sexual. Nonsexual abuse can be especially difficult to break free from because it is less obvious to those who are caught in its grip.

Consider the story of Katie, who told me, "One day my boyfriend teasingly squeezed the side of my stomach. When I asked him what he was doing, he said, 'I'm just playing with your rolls.'" Katie knew that beneath his teasing smile was the unspoken expectation that she should lose some weight if she wanted to keep him around. Horrified, she immediately went on an intense diet during which her weight dropped considerably. "My entire goal was to make him feel bad for what he said. I wanted to be frail and sick to make him pay. He wasn't listening to my voice, so I figured that maybe by physically hurting myself he would see what he had done."

Similarly, Justine suffered with feelings of low self-worth when nothing she did seemed to please her boss. Frustrated by his constant belittling, she found that controlling her diet was the only way she could feel empowered.

Like these women, we often respond to the pain of abuse by exercising unhealthy control over some aspect of our life. But when we do so, we only continue the pattern of abuse, turning inward against our very self.

Finding Healing

If you are a victim of some type of abuse, I encourage you to begin the process of healing by seeking counsel from someone you can trust. When dealing with an abusive event that occurred in our past, we often have to reopen the wound before it can be properly dressed and allowed to heal. Even though that's painful, it is an important step toward healing.

If you are currently in a situation that you feel is abusive, I encourage you to take whatever steps are necessary to remove yourself from its hold. While leaving the security of a relationship, even a damaging one, can be scary, the benefits of living freely are well worth it.

Whatever your circumstances may be, I believe that there is a loving God who will walk this road with you. Even if you feel miles away from him or are angry with him for allowing such pain in your life, I hope that you will take comfort, as I have, in the fact that he has never stopped loving you. He longs to see you live life to the fullest, and he will be there to meet you whenever you are ready.

The Role of Shame

Often the reason that past events and relationships affect us so dramatically is because, somewhere along the way, we've come to believe that there is something fundamentally wrong with who we are. Because we are ashamed of the parts of ourself that we deem unacceptable, we try to compensate by becoming what we believe is more pleasing to others. This often just compounds the problem.

For example, the bulimic's binging-and-purging pattern is inherently shaming, as is the constant deception of friends and loved ones required to maintain her secret life. For the anorexic who finds herself checked into a treatment facility, the shame of being hospitalized, along with feelings of guilt about the financial cost of her treatment, can add a new weight to an already heavy burden. And for the millions who continually battle their weight through more acceptable weight-loss methods, there can be shame in the need to even diet at all.

While these scenarios might seem obvious, those who are *successful* at controlling their weight in nonextreme ways also deal with shame. I had a hard time grasping this truth. Being thin made me feel proud, not ashamed, and so it was difficult for me to recognize that shame did indeed play a role in my issues with eating and weight. What I came to understand was that just like any other disordered eater, I was obsessed with being thin because I believed that who I was, aside from my weight, was not good enough. When someone pointed out my flaws, my internal response was, "That may be true, but at least I'm skinnier than you are!" With this defense, I avoided accepting the fact that I had a hard time loving myself as I was.

As I worked through these issues with my counselor, we slowly assembled the pieces of my past that had contributed to the way I felt about myself. The more I realized that who I was as a person was okay, the less I obsessed about how much I weighed. By understanding that I didn't have to be ashamed if I wasn't perfect or thin or beautiful, I no longer felt bound to my rigid lifestyle of dieting. This has been very freeing to me.

So What?

While we must be willing to accept responsibility for the choices we've made with regard to controlling our weight, it is helpful to recognize factors in our past that helped to shape our body image as well as our view of eating and weight.

1. What was the general attitude about weight in your home when you were growing up?

2. Describe your first memory of attaching importance to food.

3. What role do you think shame plays in your obsession with being thin?

Chapter 8

Significant Life Events

There are no little events in life, those we think of no consequence may be full of fate.

—AMELIA E. BARR, *All the Days of My Life*

Often the repercussions of traumatic events and difficulties of our early years don't show up until we reach significant transition points later in life. Dr. Donald R. Durham identifies the most significant life events as *early adolescence, leaving home, marriage, pregnancy and motherhood,* and *grief.*[1] As we move beyond our childhood dinner table and playground, these times of major change may become the pitfalls that trigger seasons of disordered eating.

Adolescence

Following our childhood years, we enter what is often the most difficult period of our lives: adolescence. In addition to ever-increasing pressure to be athletic, attractive, and popular, during adolescence we go through an extreme growth spurt that affects us physically, mentally, and emotionally. Our hormones are raging, life is frustrating, and suddenly our bodies are transforming from the straight, boylike figures we see in magazines to the fuller, curvier bodies of women.

During this critical time, the smallest of comments—however innocent—about our weight can send us reeling. Unfortunately, since many parents and siblings struggle with their own self-acceptance issues, disordered eating and negative body image are often modeled in the home. As girls then head into the changes that accompany puberty, they do so with the understanding that pursuing thinness is more important than exploring who they are.

Take Susan, a fourteen-year-old who reasons, "I just see dieting as a way to be what everyone expects me to be. If I gain too much weight, my coach will kick me off the team, and then I'll lose all my friends. I know I should eat better, but it's so hard when all my friends are as focused on weight as I am." Morgan, who is thirteen, tells me, "I sometimes notice my boyfriend checking out other girls. I need to stay thin so that he won't have any reason to dump me." Both of these girls are simply stating reality as they know it: "If you're not *thin*, you're not *in*."

Added to the pressures of perceived expectations, for many teens the emotional roller coaster of dating can lead to other unexpected troubles. Beth, who just turned sixteen, tells me, "My boyfriend recently broke up with me after we were together for three years. Even if I wanted to eat, I can't. I'm too depressed." Though Beth never worried about her weight before the breakup, her depression-induced dieting has taken on a life of its own.

It's also important to note that for teens who feel overlooked, lonely, and misunderstood, having an eating disorder in today's weight-obsessed culture can seem a logical way to find validation, community, and a sense of identity. For those who long to achieve something that will make them feel special, finding the willpower to be "successful" at dieting or starvation can seem the ultimate accomplishment. And with the abundance of Web sites that glorify and even encourage disordered eating, inspiration and incentive to begin or continue unhealthy eating practices is only a mouse click away. These sites are a haven for those wrestling with an eating disorder, and they offer honest—albeit faceless—relationship to teens who aren't finding it anywhere else.

Because of the many frustrating aspects of adolescence and the negative attitudes often displayed in the home by parents and siblings, it is no surprise that an overwhelming percentage of clinical eating disorders get their start during this period of life.

Leaving Home

The passage from being a teenager and living at home to becoming a young adult and enjoying autonomy for the first time is a significant one for most of us. Depending on our upbringing, this life event can be a joyous and exciting time or yet another daunting challenge to prove ourselves to our parents and to the world.

For many of us, college is the first time we're in control of our own diet. At home we ate whatever our parents prepared, and we didn't have to fend for ourselves. In fact, life at home was a lot easier in many ways. We knew the routine, were comfortable with the stated boundaries and curfews, and usually had a ride to wherever we needed to go.

Now we're suddenly responsible for our daily menu. And, in general, things are more difficult. The pressure to be successful at this first effort to make a name for ourselves is intense. Add to this the fact that most popular social events seem to revolve around eating and drinking, and it's no wonder that the term *Freshman Fifteen* exists. Indeed, many of us put on weight for the first time in our college years and find ourselves waging an unexpected war with food.

But while weight gain is typical, if not unwelcome, during our college years, unexpected weight loss can also trigger a problem. Consider this scenario: Ellen enters college, throws herself into her studies, and finds herself walking miles each day since she doesn't have a car. Schoolwork has taken priority over eating, and she halfheartedly eats something whenever she finds the time (and money) to have a meal. By Christmas she has unwittingly lost a few pounds. Her mother greets her at baggage claim and exclaims, "Honey, have you lost a little weight?" Ellen takes this as positive reinforcement. She's always wished she could be thinner, and now she has somehow achieved it without really trying. What was accidental weight loss has now become something she must maintain because everyone expects her to—or so she thinks.

Whatever the scenario, it is important to note that the crucial developmental step of leaving home is a potential trigger for disordered eating. In the college environment where hundreds or thousands of young people with fragile egos are thrown together, it's not surprising that eating disorders are prevalent—as many as one in five college-age women struggle with bulimia alone.[2] And chances are that those who may have struggled slightly before college will find a comfort zone in which they can allow their disordered behavior to take a turn for the worse. I mean, everybody's doing it, right?

If this is your situation right now, know that you are not alone. Others around you are battling the same feelings you are. And an increasing number of college counseling centers are becoming aware of the various types of disordered eating and can provide the help you need. If you are a parent, know that your relationship with your child during this typically difficult time can make all the difference in how he or she handles those critical first years away from home. Most important is letting your child know that you are pleased with her and love her regardless of her performance. And if she walks off that plane looking overweight (or underweight), consider how your words might have lasting implications.

Marriage

For many of us, the idea of marriage is exciting—a joyous opportunity to share life with a best friend. What we don't always realize right away is that it is also an opportunity for our habits to change, and sometimes such a transition can trigger or contribute to disordered eating.

When we're first married, we often plan meals with extra care, trying to please the taste buds of our new partner. And before we know it, we can start to put on the pounds. For those of us who already struggle with unhealthy attitudes about food, the added pressure of *having* to think more about food because we are planning meals to please someone else can exacerbate our problem.

Or perhaps we've gone through a bit of shock as we try to adjust to sharing our bed, our bathroom, our time, and our life with someone who is more complex than we thought he was. As arguments flare up, the comfort food comes out, and slowly we begin to "grow" into this relationship in more ways than one.

After a year or two we suddenly realize with alarm that we no longer fit into the cute jeans we bought to wear on our honeymoon. We start to fantasize about once again being the size we were when we married: *Everything was SO wonderful then! I was SO much more attractive. My husband must secretly be SO disap-*

pointed in me. I mean, how can he love me when I look like this? Plus, I'm not get-
ting any younger. I'd better take care of this extra weight before I'm too far gone.

And so, since none of us seems to have the patience to gradually adjust our
diet, we seek out the quickest method we can find, and we're excited to see several pounds disappear in the first week. But then that second week comes, when
all the water weight has been lost and the "real" pounds are hanging on for all
they're worth—with tiny but painfully obvious suction cups. "There simply has
to be a better way!" we lament in frustration. "Maybe I'll just skip dinner today."
So what started as an honest effort to lose extra weight turns into a binge-starve
cycle: binging then starving to make up for the binge, and then binging again to
reward ourselves for starving.

As we fight to regain control over our weight, our marital relationship begins
to feel a bit strained. For some of us, our husband becomes an unexpected judge
and jury, as my friend Cathy knows only too well. She tells me, "One night I
was getting ready for bed, and Tim looked over at me with a strange look in his
eyes. 'Maybe you should get a membership at the gym,' he said. A pang of fear
ripped through me. Suddenly I realized, *I've got to do something about my weight
if I'm going to keep my husband interested.* It really scared me."

In situations like this, a woman must somehow find the courage to accept
herself on her own terms in spite of the painful comments she may hear from
the one she loves. Her freedom lies in learning that her value is not tied to her
husband's opinion of her. Unfortunately, while easy to say, it is a painfully difficult principle to grasp.

Whether your transition into marriage is easy or difficult, the process of set-
tling into this new phase of responsibility can be a trigger for potential eating
problems.

Pregnancy

Pregnancy is a time when all the rules go out the window as our body experiences its biggest changes yet. Well-meaning friends warn us about the horrors of
hemorrhoids, varicose veins, stretch marks, and even the awful truth that our
breasts are never going to be the same perky objects of desire they once were—

and they're right! But worse than anything they can tell us is the reality that no one has to remind us about: We're going to gain weight. A lot of it.

For many women, pregnancy is the first time weight becomes an issue. Even those who have never been concerned about how they look can't help but get a little nervous as the numbers on the scale continue to climb with each passing month. And it's not just the extra pounds that are hard to accept. Equally disturbing is the strangely misshapen appearance of our body as our legs, bottom, hips, and back all expand to support our quickly expanding belly.

When we are finally delivered of our precious cargo, we enter a mind-numbing zone of sleeplessness, engorged breasts, dirty diapers, and nonstop feedings. Even though we were relieved of much of our so-called baby weight during delivery, we can't help being frustrated that our body seems to be taking its time getting rid of the remaining pounds. Some women take this all in stride. Others find themselves hating their body for the first time.

For those who are already weight conscious, pregnancy can be especially difficult. As Michelle Stacey writes in *Shape* magazine, "For the worked-out and diet-restricted, pregnancy presents the ultimate test of body control."[3] Some women react to their fears by placing even more control over their already limited diet, choosing to jeopardize a healthy pregnancy for the sake of maintaining control over their weight. Others use pregnancy as the perfect excuse to eat off-limits foods for the first time, which often leads to their gaining more weight than needed. Once the pregnancy is over, they find themselves stuck with a body they are ashamed of. In response, they either throw themselves into unhealthy eating patterns to shed the pounds, or they continue to binge in an attempt to soothe their feelings of depression, which only makes matters worse.

Though the circumstances may vary, having children is a challenging life event for every woman as well as an important contributor to the increasing numbers of late-onset eating disorders.

Grief

Another significant life event that can trigger disordered eating is grief. Jane Greer, Ph.D., writes, "When you're dealing with any kind of loss, it's an immediate blow to your self-esteem."[4] Indeed, those who have lost someone or something close to them often struggle to rediscover who they are. This process is difficult at best, and everyone seems to handle it differently.

For many of us, grieving takes away the body's natural desire for food. The pleasure associated with eating can even seem inappropriate during such times. So it is not unusual for a grieving person to lose weight unexpectedly and with little effort. And if they are complimented by well-meaning friends, many may find themselves compelled to sustain their weight loss by whatever means they can.

Others may turn to food during the grieving process to help numb the pain and fill the emptiness their loss has caused. In this case, unexpected weight gain can be disastrous, adding to the hurt and frustration they are already feeling.

Whether caused by the death of a loved one, a broken relationship, a divorce, a job change, or a move, a loss and the accompanying grief can trigger changes in our eating patterns. And since grief-causing losses often occur later in life, they can be yet another factor in late-onset disordered eating.

So What?

More than likely, you have experienced a significant life event that has triggered disordered eating and frustrating attitudes about food and your weight. You are not alone! Many women struggle with these issues at various points in their lives. But understanding the life events that often trigger seasons of disordered eating can help us move forward with making healthy choices for ourselves.

1. Which (if any) of the life events discussed in this chapter do you feel most significantly affected your body image and your view of weight and eating? Explain.

2. If you could go back in time, what would you change about the way you responded to this life event?

3. Do you see how events outside of your control might have contributed to your struggle with eating? How does that make you feel?

Chapter 9

My Body Has Betrayed Me

Weight never used to be an issue for me. Now I can't seem to keep from gaining. What's happening to me?

—BRIANNA, age thirty-four

I n addition to past events that have affected our attitudes about weight and food, unexpected physical changes can also trigger disordered eating. In conversations I've had with people about chronic dieting, we often end up discussing the fact that sometimes our body seems to betray us.

Frustrating Realities

Thyroid Problems

Last year a friend of mine found out she had cancer in her neck. A medical professional herself, she understood the importance of having the tumor removed immediately, so she underwent surgery soon after she was diagnosed. As a part of the surgery, her thyroid gland—the control center for the body's metabolism—had to be entirely removed. Not unexpectedly, following the surgery my friend began to put on weight as her body adjusted to a different metabolic rate. In my friend's case, gaining weight was not the fearful event it is for many of us, but many women do struggle with thyroid problems and with the shame and frustration they feel when their bodies seem to ignore earnest discipline and instead balloon out of control.

Diabetes

Another friend shared with me that she was incredibly frustrated with her weight and found it difficult to stop obsessing about eating because, as a diabetic, she had to maintain a strict eating schedule. Her frustration led her to struggle with all types of disordered eating, including bulimia, which only caused her to gain more weight and left her trapped in a vicious cycle.

While many of us are oblivious to the challenges of living with diabetes, millions suffer because their bodies won't function the way it was originally designed to. To learn more about the role of diabetes in eating disorders, I contacted Nicole Johnson, Miss America of 1999 and a diabetic. Offering several observations about the connection between diabetes and disordered eating, she wrote that being diabetic leads to:

1. The psychological aspect of *having* to eat, the feeling of being forced: Diabetics then feel frustrated and look for ways to find some sense of control over their eating.

2. Depression: Diabetics are more aware of their mortality and how they have to remain aware of their bodies at all times because life is fragile.

3. Societal pressure: Diabetes can sometimes lead to minor weight gain. There also can be swelling of the face and body because of the intake of insulin.

4. Fear and frustration, denial, anger, feeling like you just can't get the diabetes to cooperate, so you just give up trying and do anything you wish.[1]

Through our correspondence I also learned that many diabetics manipulate their insulin to lose weight. According to the ANRED Web site, "These folks will lose weight, but the biochemical process is particularly dangerous." Such manipulation can lead to "life-threatening organ failure and death."[2]

The truth is, a person with diabetes feels—and sometimes *is*—betrayed by her body.

Slow Metabolism

My friend Nancy is a good example of someone who simply has a slow metabolism. She can eat like a bird and still put on pounds. No matter what she does to alter her diet, she just can't seem to lose weight. It is hard to believe that some people's bodies metabolize food more slowly than the average person, but it's true. In cases like these, there is little they can do to force themselves to fit the "thin" standards of today.

Screwed-up Metabolism

One unfortunate side effect of disordered eating is that the body tries desperately to adjust to what it recognizes as starvation. As Sharlene Hesse-Biber writes, "Women who tamper with their body's natural metabolism through dieting may find they gain weight on fewer calories."[3] Once the body has time to adjust to a healthier approach to eating, the metabolism often finds its natural balance, but if you're in the midst of disordered eating, your body may surprise you with its own natural defenses.

Differing Body Types

One of my friends has a stocky build. She can't do anything about it. Even if she lost a lot of weight, she would never be as petite as some of the models she admires. This frustrates her because she often notices slim, dainty girls and wishes she could join their ranks.

Another friend of mine is petite, but her body is shaped more like a pear than an hourglass. While many women would love to have her dainty neck and petite arms, she's busy bemoaning the fact that her waist and hips are larger than she'd like them to be. Rather than focusing on discovering what kinds of clothes best complement the unique proportions of her body, she turns her energy to the latest diet or exercise routine in a desperate effort to change the unchangeable.

Both of these women have to accept the fact that no matter how much they diet, their bodies will never look like the slim, straight figures they see in magazines.

Aging

Speaking of her struggles with weight control, one woman recently wrote to me, "It certainly doesn't help that I'm getting older, and even though I haven't changed my eating, I keep gaining weight." Indeed, aging is an incredibly significant factor in feeling that our bodies are out of our control. Once women hit thirty, things begin to noticeably change, and with each year that follows, our bodies require fewer and fewer calories to maintain the same weight. As we move into middle age, hormonal changes can trigger increased mood swings, food cravings, and weight gain,[4] all of which only compound our fear of getting older. As we age, it is only natural to seek out ways to hold on to our youth, since we know that, in our culture, being older often means becoming obsolete. And since many of us don't have the cash or tolerance for plastic surgery, our weight can become something we focus on maintaining at any cost. The problem, as we'll discuss later, is that aging is inevitable, and so we are faced with the decision to make peace with it or spend the rest of our days engaged in a battle against self.

Accidents and Sickness

On January 6, 2001, my mother broke her neck in a freak car accident and is now paralyzed from the chest down. In the cruelest of ways, she has been betrayed by a body that no longer responds to her signals to move. She is stuck— a brilliant, life-loving spirit trapped in a cold casing of concrete. And for the first time, there's nothing she can do to suck in her gut. The very muscles required to do this no longer pay attention when called upon. And she must make peace with this.

Last year a friend of mine was placed on strict bed rest during the last four months of her pregnancy. Day after day she wrestled her fears, knowing that her inactivity was causing her to gain more than just baby weight. But in the interest of her child, she had no choice but to keep eating a healthy diet.

Another friend was recently diagnosed with depression and was prescribed a popular prescription medication to help even out her moods. After just a few months, she had packed nearly twenty pounds onto her petite frame. She soon realized that something in the chemical makeup of the drug was making her eat more and gain weight, but because of the seriousness of her condition, discontinuing the medication was not an immediate option.

We have no control over accidents and sickness. We could go for a walk tomorrow and be struck by a car, finding ourselves transformed instantly from perfect health to a life of painful rehab. Or we could fall ill and be forced to slow down for a while, which might cause our body to pack on the pounds. In situations like these, we must come to terms with a body that has betrayed even our best efforts at staying healthy.

So What?

When my mother was lying in the Stryker frame just hours after her accident, my only question to the doctor was, "Is her brain intact?" The rest I could deal with, but I needed to know that my mom was still there. I knew that if her brain was not damaged, she was still the same person, regardless of the body she was trapped in.

The reality is, our bodies are not always going to cooperate with our ideal of beauty and thinness. For this reason, it is crucial to come to a place where we can accept ourselves as we are—the spirit inside the body. And when our body seems to be out of our control, we can find peace by understanding that the "us" inside the body is more important than the body itself.

1.   Have you ever felt betrayed by your body? In what way?

2.   Would you be less frustrated with your body if you felt more confident about who you are as a person? Explain.

3. Looking deeper, what is it about you—your *spirit* not your body—that makes you unique?

Chapter 10

Challenging Environments

Maturity…involves thinking about one's environment and deciding what one will and won't accept.

—MARY PIPHER, *Reviving Ophelia*

For most of my life, my environment has had a great effect on me. When I arrived at Bible college at the age of sixteen, I immediately felt the pressure to prove my maturity. I carefully observed and emulated the conversation styles and mannerisms of the older students around me so that I might blend in more easily.

After I graduated and moved off campus, I found myself thrust into a society that placed a high value on material possessions. As a penniless waitress, I solved this problem by dating wealthy men. I used these relationships to surround myself with the power and influence afforded by financial excess.

When I moved to Nashville and began interacting with those in the creative community, it became apparent that the key to acceptance here was talent and marketability. So I worked hard to perfect my "look" so that I could feel relevant in an image-driven industry.

Only recently have I been able to fight the urge to meet the perceived expectations of those around me. As I've taken time to examine the power of our environment to influence our ideas about eating and food, it seems to me that certain environments foster an increased obsession with weight.

The Rich and Thin

Once in a while, when I need to be reminded of the need for this book, I'll take a trip to a trendy Nashville mall. It's one of the best places I've found to spot women who seem to believe that the size of their bodies is their most important asset. Not surprisingly, this mall happens to be in one of the more affluent parts of town. A coincidence? I doubt it.

In a short piece titled "Better Neighborhood, Worse Body Image," the June 2002 issue of *Ladies' Home Journal* noted a survey of nearly nine hundred women that indicated a connection between environment and self-esteem. Those women of average weight who lived in an affluent neighborhood had a 71 percent probability of negative body image, while their counterparts who lived in a middle-class neighborhood had a 58 percent probability.[1] That's not to say that only the wealthy struggle, but it does provoke thought.

I am continually amazed at the insatiable appetite that often accompanies abundance and success. Those who gain wealth and status seem only to desire more. As they doggedly climb the glittering social staircase, they seem oblivious to the fact that they are creating a dangerous distance between the person they feel they must become and the person they really are.

Compounding the inherent pressure of the affluent lifestyle is the idea that ultimate success requires a perfect blend of money, power, and beauty. Attaining all three can be tricky, for while money and power seem easy to attain, beauty shares herself sparingly. But for the determined individual, surgical reshaping and the art of manipulating one's body to achieve thinness can make even beauty seem like a purchasable commodity. Thus, many women of wealth willingly shell out dollars for plastic surgery, personal trainers, and trendy diets in an effort to achieve the beauty and thinness they see in the society pages of *Town and Country* magazine.

I am not suggesting that a person is certain to suffer with an eating disorder or a negative body image simply because she is wealthy, but it is important to realize that behind every richly dressed woman with perfectly applied makeup is just another human in need of love and acceptance.

Athletics and Dance

Environments that praise athleticism and perfect form are an easy place for disordered eating to thrive. Nutritionist Katherine Beals writes, "Female athletes are at a greater risk for developing disordered eating behaviors than their non-athletic counterparts."[2] It's no surprise that those involved in sports feel an immense amount of pressure to sacrifice their health in order to "make weight" for the team.

For those who have never struggled with unhealthy eating, being in an environment that glorifies fitness can trigger unexpected weight issues. Beals also notes that sports emphasizing leanness often attract those who already have eating disorders, offering them an outlet to either justify or hide their behavior.[3]

Those with a passion for dance face similar challenges. While athletes equate thinner with faster, better, and stronger, dancers see being thin as an essential component in mastering the graceful and powerful movements associated with their craft. My friend Stacy explains the struggle: "I know I'm not fat, but when I'm rehearsing, it's hard not to notice the other girls who are thinner than I am." Surrounded by mirrors that reflect every angle, she has a hard time avoiding obsessing about her body. "I sometimes don't even think about my dancing," she tells me. "I'm too busy looking at everyone else and comparing my body with theirs."

In such highly perfectionistic environments, even the tiniest traces of body fat are seen as unacceptable and can trigger or exacerbate disordered eating. So what is one to do? These activities can be healthy developmental and recreational outlets; must we now consider them off-limits? Again, we have to go back to the issue of balance. If you are able to balance your dreams of being a world-class runner with the importance of being healthy, then by all means train hard and run the race. And if dancing brings you joy that overcomes the pressure to look skeletal, then give it your all. But if these activities become either an excuse or a trigger for disordered eating, it is important to stop for a moment and consider the price you may pay.

Modeling and Fashion

Charis, a young aspiring model, tells me, "I went to a photo shoot last week, and the photographer said I was too fat—that I was ruining his pictures." Another model-in-training sits beside her, gaunt eyes and pale skin betraying the fact that she's been starving herself for weeks. "It's just the way it is," she says, matter-of-factly. "If you want to be a successful model, you've got to be more than a pretty face. You've got to be very, very thin." And she's right, at least according to statistics.

Today the average model is five feet eleven inches tall and weighs only 117 pounds.[4] And while the influence of such thin imaging can make it difficult for the average woman to feel good about her body, models themselves struggle under the pressure to stay thin.

"The fashion world isn't an environment where health is necessarily encouraged," says Carre Otis, a highly successful model who spent several years starving herself and abusing drugs to stay thin. Now at a healthier place physically, mentally, emotionally, and spiritually, Carre notes, "I used to measure how I felt based on what size jean I wore, how skinny I was. Now I see myself in terms of health."[5] But while Carre has found peace with accepting her body at a healthier weight, many models would rather die than be considered anything but model thin. So they spend their days denying their bodies of that which brings true contentment in favor of meeting unrealistic, airbrushed ideals of beauty.

The Creative World

As a creative person who has spent many years working in the entertainment industry, I have personally experienced the insecurity, frustration, and conflict that often exist within the creative community. It's not that those who have been blessed with some gifting or talent always lead tragic lives, but often they seem to face more trials than the average person. I imagine much of this has to do with the fact that those with highly active brains can overanalyze things to the point of distress. Another key factor is that many creative types tend to think that they must achieve a certain image to fit into the artistic community. Unfortunately, this so-called image is difficult to maintain for several reasons.

First, in many creative circles you're only as good as your last success (or failure), which is a precarious place to live. Second, many of us who are creative esteem aesthetic beauty so highly that we can find it difficult to accept imperfection in ourselves or in those around us. Understandably, perfecting our body through dieting and disordered eating can seem a worthwhile goal in this environment.

Those who find a public platform for their gift face even greater challenges. Now, in addition to seeking acceptance and community among their peers, they are also judged openly by the media according to ever-changing and often-unrealistic standards of beauty and weight. And while many of them can probably afford the latest weight-control programs and high-end cosmetic techniques, by the time they reach the ideals set for them by the public, they are dehydrated, demoralized, and creatively stifled. The energy they once channeled into honing their craft has been redirected into struggling to meet the expectations of others—and their self-esteem and inner spirit are torn down as a result.

To be creative, one needs a healthy balance of work and play, relationship and solitude, joy and sorrow, praise and criticism. And yes, nutrition and exercise. These all go hand in hand. When we starve any of these areas, its counterpart only grows stronger. We lose the benefit of balance, and our ability to create is stifled.

Don't Discount the Genes

As my mom has gently reminded me, all of this talk about environment needs to be balanced with the fact that some of us have a genetic predisposition to unhealthy behaviors, which can be triggered by certain environments. Indeed, much attention is currently being given to discovering whether there is an actual genetic link in eating disorders, particularly anorexia.[6]

In addition to the complexities of our genetic makeup, we should also take into account the unique aspects of our personality when considering how environmental factors can trigger unhealthy behavior. For example, I am a highly achievement-driven person. When placed in a performance-oriented situation, I tend to throw myself into workaholic mode so that I can exceed the expectations of my superiors. Conversely, someone with a more easygoing personality might be willing to head home once the day is done, knowing that his or her value does not depend on accomplishing the impossible. For this person, a performance-driven environment is not as unhealthy.

What makes you tick? Are you compulsive or calculating? Is it difficult for you to be in a room with other women without feeling that you don't measure up? Do social occasions bring out the part of you that leaves no room for mistake?

By exploring the unique characteristics of our personality and genetic makeup in relation to our environment, we can understand more about what is behind our disordered eating behavior.

So What?

When it comes to choosing our environment, there's nothing wrong with being surrounded by people who are focused on material and temporal things, as long as their focus doesn't blur our own. The key to true freedom is to realize that just because something is important to someone else, it doesn't mean we have to live according to their value system. We have the right to choose which values we want to preserve as our own.

1. What aspects of your environment seem to trigger your obsession with weight control?

2. If you were able to move somewhere entirely different, would this solve your problem? Why or why not?

3. What factors in your natural genetic makeup seem to contribute to your obsessions (i.e., perfectionistic, high-strung, etc.)?

The Hollywood Effect

I wish people would be more honest about how much work it takes to look the way women in Hollywood do.

—Natalie Raitano, actress

I started undereating, overexercising, pushing myself too hard, and brutalizing my immune system.

—Courtney Thorne-Smith, speaking of her chronic dieting while on *Ally McBeal*

Many of us would have an easier time accepting the natural size of our bodies if not for the constant reminders of perfection coming from Hollywood. Indeed, Hollywood plays a dramatic—and often self-debilitating—role in promoting an image that is increasingly unattainable. In addition to the devastating effects on the general public, this unhealthy focus on thinness has perpetuated a vicious cycle that is beginning to haunt Hollywood itself, as those in the acting community willingly sacrifice their health and well-being to achieve the latest standard of thinness. Each success sets the bar even higher—and the acceptable dress size even lower. If you think all is well in Tinseltown, think again.

Incredible Shrinking Stars

A phenomenon of revolutionary proportions is happening in Hollywood: The stars are shrinking. Consider some of the actresses hailed these days for their undeniably thin bodies: Lara Flynn Boyle, Ashley Judd, Helen Hunt, Debra

Messing, Meg Ryan, Christina Ricci. All of these stars were noticeably more filled out in the earlier days of their careers. And they are not alone. At the beginning of taping for *Frasier*, Jane Leeves (Daphne) was a woman of average size. But by the 2000 season, she was praised for her ultrathin figure by the admittedly weight-obsessed Joan Rivers, who awarded her the Golden Hanger Award for her impeccable style.

And when we all met Jennifer Aniston (Rachel) for the first time on *Friends*, it was more than just her trendy hairstyle that we wanted to copy. With her fuller girlish figure, she was a beautiful example of how curves are definitely sexy. Though admittedly curvier than her castmates, Aniston seemed to be the public's favorite "friend," gracing the cover of numerous magazines and landing starring roles in feature films.

But by the late 1990s, Aniston's weight started dropping significantly. Before long she had officially joined the ranks of the ultrathin, much to the delight of the media—and the dismay of her own personal trainer.[1] Aniston's costar Courtney Cox seemed to follow suit, her weight noticeably dropping until she was a mere shadow of the startling beauty we admired in Jim Carrey's film *Ace Ventura: Pet Detective*. Recently, both women have seemed to stop shrinking, but their weight continues to be noticed and commented on by the media. And while much of the attention they receive praises them for their thinness, I imagine that the close scrutiny of the press has a powerful effect on the way they see their bodies and their weight.

It is disheartening to see these and other truly beautiful women fall victim to the cultlike practices of the weight obsessed. They trade in their happiness for a life of rules, restrictions, and self-denial in pursuit of an ideal that continues to shrink. So how have we gotten to this point?

Prime-Time Power

While image and success have always gone hand in hand in Hollywood, this trend toward the ultrathin seems fairly recent. The first time I noticed the pervasiveness of such thin imaging was in the midnineties on *Melrose Place*. The show's stars, most notably Josie Bisset and Heather Locklear, set a new standard for sexy with their unusually slim bodies. One scene that sticks out in my mind was when Heather's character Amanda was trying on a dress and said to her boyfriend, "Bring me the 2." With her simple statement, a clothing size many of us had once considered too small became something to shoot for. Actually having a number attached to the model of beauty we observed each week on the show gave us a tangible goal for our weight-loss efforts. And since most of the show's stars were quite well endowed in the chest, their unusually thin bodies didn't alarm us, since bustier women often have the appearance of being healthy even when the rest of their body betrays a lack of nutrition. So as we became desensitized to the image of ultrathin women on *Melrose Place,* the stage was perfectly set for the introduction of a new show that would single-handedly transform the skeletal image of anorexia into an object of desire.

Ally McBeal

With the 1997 premier of *Ally McBeal,* the show's star, Calista Flockhart, spawned a whole new ideal of perfection in Hollywood. Unlike her predecessors on *Melrose Place,* who continued to display the sex appeal of womanly curves— if only in their chest—Flockhart broke the tried-and-true Hollywood mold by presenting a new ideal of the frail, quirky, and clever "little girl." Not only was she startlingly thin, but her chest was nearly flat, as if to convey on some level the idea of a budding adolescent thrown into the games and chaos of an adult world. Everything Flockhart did both on- and offscreen seemed to be praised and admired. Even her highly talented castmates couldn't seem to achieve the same level of intrigue that drew us to the delicate picture of Flockhart's youthful beauty.

Soon after the show's first season, several publications began commenting on what seemed to be the suddenly plummeting weight of actresses in Hollywood. In just a few short months the average dress size of actresses dropped from an already slender 6 or 4 to a 2 or even a 0.[2]

Ally McBeal is now off the air, but the show's effects are not so easily canceled. Of course, *Ally McBeal* isn't the only show guilty of promoting the emaciated look, but it certainly seems to have set the pace for follow-up performances by several actresses. The good news is that even Hollywood is starting to pay attention to the reality of this unhealthy obsession.

The Backlash

In response to the ever-increasing demands to lose weight, many actresses have begun to pay a noticeable price. In fact, the weight-conscious environment of *Ally McBeal* became particularly debilitating for the cast. In 2000, *Ally*'s Portia de Rossi admitted to Britain's *Sunday Express,* "I got on the Hollywood bandwagon… Unfortunately, I got to a weight where I just didn't look good anymore."[3] She went on to say that she put some weight back on once she realized she had gone too far.

De Rossi's former castmate Courtney Thorne-Smith shared a similar experience and even chose to leave the show to take better care of herself. She told *US Weekly* that working alongside one of the thinnest actresses in Hollywood (Flockhart) severely undermined her self-esteem. "I started undereating, over-exercising, pushing myself too hard and brutalizing my immune system," she said, speaking of the intense pressure to lose weight.[4]

And these women are not alone. A simple viewing of Joan Rivers's Red Carpet report will bring into clear view the many celebrities suffering physically, mentally, and emotionally from the pressure to fit in. And while Hollywood is probably not going to stop placing a premium on thinness, it seems to have recognized that not only is the public at large hungry for more realistic body types, but even the celebrities are crying out for a change.

In September 2002 actress and children's author Jamie Lee Curtis bravely challenged the Hollywood ideal when she posed for *More* magazine without makeup, hairstyling, or attractive lighting, wearing only a sports bra and unflattering spandex briefs. Her purpose was to challenge the myth of Hollywood perfection she had admittedly helped perpetuate. In the article, aptly titled "True Thighs," Jamie openly discussed the truth about her body. "I don't have great thighs," she said. "I have very big breasts and a soft, fatty little tummy. Glam Jamie, the perfect Jamie…it's such a fraud." And the photo backs up her statement. Gone are the rock-hard thighs and flat tummy she's always been associated with. In their place is the normal, healthy body of a forty-three-year-old woman. But in spite of the untoned tummy and not-so-thin thighs that the photo betrays, most surprising about the image is Jamie's unabashed take-me-as-I-am smile, suggesting that accepting one's body brings a great sense of relief.[5]

Curtis isn't the only actress going public about accepting her body on her own terms. Téa Leoni, who has purposely kept some of the weight she gained during her first pregnancy, says, "I'm much happier with my body now. If I'm not rail-thin enough for Hollywood, I'm sure they'll let me know, and I'll be glad to leave."[6] Commenting on the pressure to lose weight after the birth of her daughter, Kate Winslet says, "I shall always be the curvy Kate that everybody knows."[7] It is the positive attitude of self-acceptance projected by stars like these that gives credence to so many of us who are frustrated with an ideal of beauty that we know we can't achieve.

Even Hollywood executives are adding their influence to the cry for "normal" body types. Says *The Grinch* producer Brian Grazer, "I don't want the actresses I work with to get too thin—I just don't like the way that looks."[8] Fran Bascom, casting director for NBC's *Days of Our Lives,* shares a similar view: "I look for the best actor for the role… After all, fans come in all sizes, and they can relate to someone who isn't a size 2."[9]

Perhaps in recognition of the truth that fans indeed come in all sizes, in October 2002 HBO aired the body-confident movie *Real Women Have Curves,* which portrays normal-size women who find relief and humor in their less-than-perfect bodies.[10] And more than a few new television shows for the 2002 fall season featured actresses who are a more accurate representation of the average woman.

But while some media outlets seem to have a renewed interest in presenting what is "real," we must remember that Hollywood's very existence depends upon providing the element of fantasy so many of us desire. And what greater fantasy is there than to have a perfectly gorgeous body?

So What?

Hollywood plays a dramatic and often self-debilitating role in promoting an image that is increasingly unattainable. But while many stars choose to risk their health and well-being in order to get a part, more and more women are crying

out for permission to eat, permission to look like a woman, permission to be
who they are. We all deserve this freedom.

1. Think of the television shows that make you feel dissatisfied with your
    body or weight…the shows that give you incentive to keep losing weight.
    List as many as you can.

2. Name a celebrity you admire who is not ultrathin.

3. How would you feel about your body if everyone on television were at
    least a size 8 or 10? Explain.

Prayer

*God, please reveal to me the ways in which my human nature
contributes negatively to the way I feel about myself.*

*Give me the strength to forgive those who have been unkind
to me or who have treated me unfairly in the past.*

*Help me make wise decisions when it comes to evaluating my environment
and its effect on my self-image and eating habits.*

I want to live in freedom.

PART 3

WHAT KEEPS US TRAPPED?

When I was a young girl, watching my mother go through episodes of binging and purging often frustrated me. I couldn't understand why she continued living what I knew was an incredibly unhealthy and unhappy lifestyle. I remember thinking one night that I should just go to her and say, "Mom, don't you know you're killing yourself?" At which point I imagined her saying, "Why, I never really thought about it that way. You're right—I should stop this!" But we never had that conversation, and I'm quite sure it wouldn't have made a difference if we had.

Years later, when the tables were turned and I was the one obsessed with eating and weight, my mom probably felt the same way I had earlier. In fact, for more than ten years both of my parents made comments and questioned me about the way I was eating, but I remained intent on continuing my lifestyle. It was "working" for me, and that was all I really cared about.

If you've just figured out that your obsession with dieting is actually working against you rather than in your best interests, you might be wondering why it's so hard to change the way you've been living.

The truth is, there are many reasons why perfectly logical people remain in situations that are unhealthy. In this section we'll get at the heart of many of these reasons.

We Don't Know We're in It

It's been a couple weeks since I finally decided I was sick and tired of this game. Somehow something just clicked. I realized that the last eleven years of my life have not been my own. I have sacrificed them willingly to appease this demon inside. Somehow, moving into a home for the first time, being more in touch with nature around me, and realizing a forgotten desire to be active have served as catalysts to jerk me into a different perspective on this whole thing.

I am tired of being the weak, frail waif. There was a time (most of the past eleven years) when "waif" was all I aspired to achieve. It's a sick thing, this thinking pattern. I guess what's most surprising to me is that only now is the light going off for me. I've only just begun to realize that this is *not* a good thing for me. This does *not* give me an edge. Rather, it makes me too weak and faint to enjoy life to its fullest. So, somehow, I'm realizing that I'm determined to beat this thing. I know it won't be easy, but for once I really want to get rid of the monster…

Why did I just now realize this?

—FROM MY JOURNAL, May 31, 2000

It's hard to get out of a cage if we don't know we're in it. Most of us remember the Looney Toons episode where Elmer Fudd puts Bugs Bunny in a pot and slowly heats the water. For a while Bugs is quite comfortable, exulting in what he thinks is a nice warm bath. Suddenly he senses that something is wrong—things have gotten too hot for him. Because it started out as an innocent bath, he didn't realize he was in a trap until it was almost too late. But in true Bugs fashion, he makes his way out just in time.

Many of us aren't so lucky. While Bugs's trap seems obvious, ours has been masked by a culture that praises dieting, and it has been ignored by a medical and professional community whose focus is on more extreme eating disorders and the increasing problem of obesity.

For some of us, the ability to think objectively and logically about our lifestyle has been further compromised by our refusal to feed our bodies and brains the nutrients they need to serve us well. I experienced this when I went through my anorexic stage. After months of depriving myself of essential fats that help the brain function properly, I found I had a hard time distinguishing fact from fiction. When people said I looked too thin, I truly thought they were crazy. Looking back at photos, I am stunned to see how unhealthy I looked during that time.

But as I made my way out of this and other more obvious phases of disordered eating, I came to believe that the way I was living was perfectly normal. And I worked hard to convince everyone else of it too.

Living in Denial

For many years when my father and mother would make comments about my low weight, I would reply, "I don't have an eating disorder. I just watch what I eat." It's not that I was just saying this to get them off my back. I honestly believed my own excuses. I would dispute this point many times over the years, sometimes just for the sake of argument. I couldn't understand why no one ever seemed to believe me.

I was in denial.

What is denial, and why do we choose to live in it? To me, denial is a buffer between what I want and why I shouldn't have it. It's like refusing to look at my budget before going shopping, so that I can ignore the fact that I shouldn't really be spending any money. Denial doesn't change the balance in my bank account, but it temporarily removes the guilt of spending more money than I probably should.

Denial is also a popular pain-avoidance tool. For example, those who have suffered abuse often deny that anything has happened. To accept what has happened would mean that something needs to be done about it, and that could be as painful as the event itself.

In the same way, many of us who chronically diet deny that we're obsessed. We deny that our eating habits are anything but health conscious. But in denying the truth, we unwittingly deny ourselves of other things, such as the joy of eating without feeling guilty…or the opportunity to invest our time and energy in deepening our relationships with friends and loved ones…or the satisfaction of living life to the fullest.

Living in denial is never a positive move. The woman in denial of an abusive relationship sees the bruises on her face as an indication that she is not good enough. The alcoholic in denial of his addiction becomes an island in his own home, too numb to recognize the devastating effects of his behavior on those around him. The partner in denial of an unhealthy relationship only pushes away the opportunity to find a true soul mate.

When we are in denial, truth cannot touch us. It isn't until we choose to face reality that we will start to realize the truths that can free us.

So What?

Coming out of denial and embracing the truth is a difficult but important first step. By choosing to recognize the ways in which our obsession with dieting has trapped us, we give ourselves incentive to reconsider our views on eating and weight.

1. Do you see your disordered eating as a trap? Why or why not?

2. What are some of your most common responses when someone suggests that you might not be eating right?

3. What would be the scariest thing about admitting that you've become obsessed with weight and eating?

Making Choices out of Fear

If I gain weight people will look down on me, not respect me.

—ALLISON, age forty-six

While denial can keep us from realizing we're trapped in a lifestyle of unhealthy eating, it is fear that most often stands between us and freedom from the thin cage. For even when we become more aware of how we're trapped, we might be too afraid to find a way out.

The Fears That Drive Us

"What If I Gain Weight?"

Fear has the power to paralyze. Politicians who fear losing votes may back away from the very issues that inspired them to run for election. CEOs, in fear of losing their "golden parachute," may ignore questionable accounting practices. In the same way, many of us have become paralyzed by our fear of losing control over our weight.

In her July 2001 article in *Elle* magazine, writer Andrea Morris discusses how fear was a major factor in her own subclinical eating disorder. She writes, "Despite all the evidence that my health and state of mind will benefit from improved eating, my biggest concern is whether it will make me gain weight."[1]

Indeed, it is scary to leave a tried-and-true method of weight control and trust the nonmanipulated abilities of our body. We don't know for sure that we're going to like the results. And what if we're actually destined to be heavy? What then?

When taking steps to overcome this fear, we must first consider how many things we've come to believe are dependent on our weight. Things like:

- respect
- attention
- importance/relevance
- beauty
- love
- control
- sex appeal
- self-confidence
- self-esteem
- opportunities
- our career
- the ability to see our dreams come true
- security
- social standing
- friends

Why is it that we believe these things are contingent on what size we wear? Could it be that, like the politician and the CEO, our fear has paralyzed us and kept us from the truth?

For Andrea Morris, facing her fears made them less powerful. After nervously agreeing to her nutritionist's suggestion that she eat six small healthy meals a day, thus regulating her blood sugar and regularly giving her body the nourishment it needed, she notes, "I am sleeping decently, feeling less edgy, not craving chocolate…and my clothes are loose. While I still have my bad body-image days, they come less frequently, and I can move on fairly quickly."[2]

Morris's story is a great example of the freedom that is found in facing our fears. It also reinforces the fact that our bodies will generally regulate themselves as long as we feed them properly. In fact, by eating right, our blood-sugar levels are stabilized, which prevents our body from entering starvation mode, during which calories are stored by the body as fat instead of being used as energy. Only by giving our body what it needs can we be assured that it will rest at its normal weight. Of course, we must be prepared to accept that our body's normal rest-ing weight and our ideal picture of thin might be different, but even this becomes easier when we face our fear of weight gain. As nutritionist Jill Malden explains, "When you keep blood-sugar levels stable, you'll feel and sleep better; when you feel better you're less obsessive."[3]

"People Expect Me to Be Thin"

Time and again I hear from women who say that even if they themselves feel okay about gaining weight, their fear of what others expect prevents them from reclaiming their rightful body. My conversations have led me to a few truths that challenge this misperception:

1. Most people do *not* expect us to be as thin as we think we must be.
2. Some people may always expect us to be different than we are.
3. Trying to live up to someone else's expectations is usually achieved only at the expense of our own desires.

It is important to realize that we can only be happy when we live true to who we are. In the end, most people will love us more for learning to do so.

"I Don't Want to Be Labeled"

For some of us, the fear of being labeled is just as great as the fear of gaining weight. The very idea of admitting that we struggle with disordered eating represents failure to us, and since we've done such a good job removing the obvious signs of failure from our lives, why should we concede in front of God and everyone now?

If this concern sounds familiar, I'm right there with you. Even now my mother has to remind me that at one point I actually did fit all the criteria for anorexia, something I still hate to admit. I don't know why this is so hard for me—you'd think that now that I'm willing to air my dirty laundry for the world to see, I would at least feel comfortable with the terminology. But I still find myself fighting it. I never wanted to be anorexic, and I can't believe that I ever fit that classification—but I did.

As I've begun to talk more openly about my struggle with disordered eating, I've discovered that one good thing about our culture is that we live in an age where differences are embraced. And while there are always going to be those who would rather believe that everything (and everyone) is perfect and without blemish, more and more of us are supporting honesty and forgiving failure.

Of course, honesty gets more difficult when it gets personal. We appreciate Susan's honesty about her drinking problem and Steve's boldness in admitting his struggle with pornography, but we feel that our problem is much worse than theirs. "I could never admit to having an eating disorder," we tell ourselves. "What would everyone think?"

But just like all the other little lies we've been fed while in the cage, the idea that people are suddenly going to turn tail and run once they know our secret is often far from true. The truth is, most people will actually be relieved to know that you, like them, don't have it all together. Not to mention the fact that for many of us, our secret is, in reality, only a secret to us. With more and more people becoming aware of unhealthy dieting practices, don't be surprised if they're not shocked when you come clean.

"I Must Be Perfect"

Many of us view perfectionism as a desirable quality rather than the fear-based flaw that it is. Think about it: Has it ever bothered you to be called a perfectionist? Do we not find ourselves demurely shrugging off the suggestion with a modest smile, saying something like, "Well, I just like to make sure things are done right"? Truth be told, we're *proud* to be called perfectionists, because it makes us feel indispensable, worthy of our paycheck, and deserving of the admiration of others. But isn't perfectionism really just an attempt to eliminate the possibility of rejection?

If we're really honest, we must admit that for most of us who struggle to accept ourselves the way we are, perfectionism is an easy trap to fall into. We believe that if we could just perfect *something* about ourselves, we would finally be undeniably worthy of love and acceptance. Since our external appearance is our most notable attribute, it seems only natural to focus on perfecting our body.

The problem is that the closer we get to whichever standard of perfection we seek, the less satisfied we are. As I lost the weight I had gained in college, being thin was no longer enough for me. Now I wanted my hair to be perfect, so I spent hundreds of dollars to attain the right color weaves and cuts. And what were a perfect body and perfect hair without perfect clothes? So I went shopping and racked up burdensome credit-card bills in my search for the perfect outfit—hoping that the right clothes would prevent others from seeing my flawed self. Soon even this wasn't enough, and my drive for perfection extended beyond my physical appearance to the overall image I wished to project to anyone watching. It now became important to make sure I was hanging out with the right people. In conversations I made every effort to laugh at all the appropriate places, and I always tried to make sure I was prepared with clever responses at every turn. My need for perfection permeated everything I did. No detail was too small to be scrutinized under the microscope.

The difficult part about seeking perfection is that everyone has a different idea of what true perfection is. What is perfect in the eyes of one person may seem flawed to someone else. And even if we think we know what someone else considers perfect, our dependence on that person's opinion only weakens our ability to love ourselves as we are. So where do we go from here?

"It all comes down to learning your own value, I guess," writes Michelle, a twenty-something professional who has battled her own negative self-image. "I have come to understand that perfection isn't a productive lifestyle and that I'm the only one who considers myself a success if and only if I have it *all* together *all* the time."

So, as we leave the nonproductive pursuit of perfection, we have the opportunity to switch our focus to seeking excellence instead. Dr. Donald Durham offers the following distinction between the two: "Excellence acknowledges that there is always room for improvement, but it doesn't demand it *now*."[4] Indeed, this gives us room to be human.

So What?

Fear is not a positive motivator. Too often it can paralyze us, preventing us from making choices that would bring us true joy and contentment.

1. We face many fears when we decide to make our escape from the thin cage. Which fears do you struggle with? Finish this sentence: "I'm afraid that if I gain weight, I will lose…"

2. Does it surprise you to consider that perfectionism is based in fear? How has a desire for perfection played into your unhealthy eating habits?

3. If fear were not a factor, do you think you would continue your unhealthy lifestyle? Explain.

We're Addicted

Essentially, sufferers of eating disorders are psychologically addicted to weight control.

—LINDY BEAM, editor of *Beyond Appearances*

E ven when we decide to face our fears about changing the way we eat, we must reckon with yet another powerful force: addiction.

Some of the well-meaning people who encouraged me to "just eat a little" could not understand that not only was I not interested in making them happy by stopping my dieting, but I was actually addicted to my lifestyle—physically, mentally, and emotionally. And just like other addictions, this one was going to take some serious effort to break.

Physical Addictions

The physical effects of dieting and disordered eating impact more than just our weight. Those who struggle with disordered eating normally suffer from some sort of physical addiction to food. Following are just a few of the ways a physical addiction can play into our struggles:

Sugar, Flour, and Mood-Altering Foods

I first became aware of the influence of sugar on our body and brain when I read my mother's journals years ago. Intent on finding the elusive key to freedom from her bulimia, my mom had discovered a consistent connection between her intake of sugar and her out-of-control appetite. For example, she found that she would feel calmer and was less likely to binge if she chose pretzels instead of a candy bar for a snack.

Years after reading my mother's notes, I discovered this same connection in my own eating struggles. When I ate foods that were high in sugar, I seemed to crave more—even though I knew I didn't really want the sugar in my system. After a few days of avoiding candy and other high-sugar foods, I would feel calmer and less out of control.

In their book *Why Can't I Stop Eating?* recovering food addict Debbie Danowski and medical doctor Pedro Lazaro point out that, according to many studies, "Sugar is one of the most physiologically addictive substances."[1] (They go on to say that the average American consumes more than 151 pounds of sugar per year!)

Many of us who watch what we eat may think we've done well to remove excess sweets from our diet when in fact the opposite may be true. For example, as we discussed in chapter 4, chronic dieters often try to maintain a low-fat or fat-free diet. What these dieters may not realize is that "in many cases, low-fat foods contain more sugar than 'regular' ones to provide enhanced flavor."[2] Because of this, low-fat eaters often end up eating larger quantities of sugar than they realize, which only makes them hungrier.

As powerful as sugar may be, it is not the only culprit when it comes to food addictions. Other common ingredients such as white flour, caffeine, wheat, and even fat have been referred to as mood-altering substances, all of which can cause a physiological addiction that can be even stronger than that of sugar. If this is true, then the bagel we're eating for breakfast instead of scrambled eggs and sausage can actually make us want to eat more. Similarly, the caffeine we're drinking to help stimulate our energy may also increase our appetite.

The Serotonin Connection

The powerful effect that sugar and other foods can have on us often has to do with the way they impact our serotonin levels. Serotonin is the chemical in our brain that regulates our mood and helps our minds focus. When our serotonin level is high, we feel calm and happy and can handle greater amounts of stress.

But when our serotonin level drops, so does our mood, and we can become edgy, distracted, and even depressed.

Because certain foods such as carbohydrates can momentarily boost our serotonin level, we often associate eating them with feeling good. When our serotonin level drops, we can find ourselves craving the very foods we're trying to avoid. For those of us who obsess about what we eat, this addictive urge can trigger frustrated binging followed by even more dieting. This only compounds the problem, as Julia Ross, author of *The Diet Cure,* explains: "As [dieters] eat less, their serotonin levels fall farther, increasing [their] obsession with under-eating."[3]

Ross explains that, among other things, low serotonin levels can contribute to a loss of self-esteem and to obsessive behaviors. Because of this, "Extreme dieting is actually the worst way to try to raise self-esteem, because the brain can only deteriorate further and become more self-critical as it starves."[4]

As the benefits of serotonin have been explored and are better understood, serotonin-regulating drugs such as Prozac and Zoloft have grown in popularity. But the link between obsessive dieting and the resulting low serotonin levels is not often discussed.

The fact is, for many of us, simply changing our diet to include more foods that contain tryptophan (the amino acid that creates serotonin) would help us break away from our addictive and obsessive behaviors. And unlike prescription drugs, most of which don't actually create *more* serotonin, naturally occurring tryptophan can give us the benefits of increased serotonin levels without the frustrating side effects of medications. (For more information on this topic, I highly recommend Julia Ross's book.)

Physically Addicted to Not Eating?

On the opposite end of food addiction is the fact that if we stop eating regular-size meals, our stomachs can shrink, making it physically difficult to eat more, even when we really want to. I experienced this when I first started breaking free from chronic dieting. After years of eating small portions, my stomach had a hard time adjusting to the normal amounts of food I was trying to add to my diet. This would often lead to discomfort, cramping, and even diarrhea. In a way, my body was physically addicted to *not* eating. Even though I wanted to eat more to be healthier, it was very difficult for me to go against what my body was telling me. For the weight obsessed, overcoming a lack of appetite can be just as difficult as breaking an addiction to certain foods.

Mental and Emotional Addictions

While physical addictions are difficult to contend with, many of us have grown equally addicted to the mental and emotional "benefits" of our lifestyle. Following are a few of the ways our minds can keep us locked into our obsessive patterns.

"I'm Enjoying This Ride"

The primary addiction I faced was the mental rush I felt when I realized I was the thinnest woman in the room. During this time I was incredibly addicted to the attention I got from others, even though I realize now that some of the glances I assumed to be admiring were actually troubled or even disgusted by my overly thin body. But in my mind, life would have been over if I had no longer received this attention. Sharlene Hesse-Biber tells us, "Thinness gives women access to a number of important resources: feelings of power, self-confidence, even femininity; male attention or protection; and the social and economic benefits that can follow."[5] In this context, it's easy to understand how one might become addicted to the benefits of maintaining a thin body.

Take my friend Meredith. She is continually told by admiring women that they wish they had a body like hers. And she has no shortage of male friends who regularly shower her with compliments. With each approving glance, Meredith becomes more and more addicted to the looks she receives by being a thin and attractive person.

"If I gained weight, I would hate my life," she told me one evening over coffee.

"But aren't you tired of always obsessing about what you weigh?" I asked her.

"Sometimes," she admitted. "But being thin makes me feel good. I don't want to live without that feeling."

Another woman wrote to me, saying, "When I was heavier, I always felt so masculine. I feel more feminine now—like a delicate flower that needs to be protected and cherished." She went on to say that her husband seems to fawn over her more now that she's thinner. And while she recognizes that she thinks about eating and weight "more often than is probably healthy," she is unwilling to part with what she deems a central part of true femininity—being small.

"Controlling My Diet Makes Me Feel Secure"

While many women are addicted to the benefits of being thin, another friend of mine has become addicted to the sense of security she finds in the rigidity of her lifestyle. Because she is the type of person who thrives on order and structure, she honestly believes that her life would come crashing down around her if she dared to be more flexible with her eating habits. Indeed, for those of us who are addicted to the feeling of being in control, the idea of relaxing our self-imposed diet rules flies in the face of protecting what we've looked to for our comfort and security.

"I Need the Release"

Yet another addictive element is the feeling of release that some find in the disordered eating process. For example, those who purge by throwing up often feel a sense of euphoria immediately following their purge. And while this feeling is quickly replaced with guilt, shame, frustration, and fear, the momentary euphoria can become addictive for many people. For others who find their comfort in food, binging can momentarily bring them relief in times of great stress. Similarly, for those who are suffering from deep pain in their life, binging, purging, and starving can seem like a coping mechanism for their pain in much the same way that a "cutter" finds relief by slashing her arms. Unfortunately, the pain they are trying to soothe is only compounded by their efforts, and they find themselves trapped in an addictive cycle they can't seem to break.

So What?

Determining the ways in which addiction contributes to our unhealthy lifestyle is a key step in breaking free from our destructive patterns.

1. Do you often find yourself thinking about food and wanting to eat even if you've already eaten? Give an example.

2. Does it seem that the more you eat, the more you want? Conversely, does it seem that the less you eat, the less you want? Write down a few examples of this.

3. What do you think you are most addicted to when it comes to your unhealthy eating (i.e., "being thin and getting attention from others," "feeling like I'm in control")?

Good Help Is Hard to Find

Years ago when I first admitted I had a problem, I went to a well-known treatment facility in California.... I went along with their diagnosis and treatment and of course got nothing out of it because they didn't understand my problem at all.

—SARAH, age thirty-five

I just wish they would stop asking me what I'm eating and how much I weigh now and get to the heart of my problem—my disgust with myself as a person.

—CHRIS, age twenty-seven

Changing the ideas behind our behavior requires taking a journey into the events and experiences that have contributed to what we believe about ourselves. Once we are ready to take this journey, there is nothing more disheartening than not being able to find the right person to guide us toward healing. Time after time I hear from people who have ended up with therapists and counselors who just don't seem to help them. But even though these women know they're not getting what they need, they often feel too guilty to seek out a new therapist. So they end up wasting money and time and don't get any closer to resolving their issues.

The good news is that thousands of people have found the key to unlocking their cage through the help of a psychologist or counselor. It takes time to establish a fruitful relationship with a therapist, so it's important to give that relationship a chance before you move on. As you consider whether a particular counselor is right for you, however, you may want to keep the following observations in mind.

Clinical Approaches Sometimes Miss the Point

As we discussed in chapter 2, when a person does not fit the textbook classification for anorexia, bulimia, or binge eating, the professional community is often unsure how to treat the disorder. This is what happened to me when I first sought out psychological care for my problem.

As I explained to the therapist what was going on—that I would sometimes skip meals one day but eat quite normally the next day—I could tell that she was searching for an appropriate response to my problem. After only two sessions, she wrote me a prescription for Prozac, which had recently been shown to be helpful in treating some eating disorders. Honestly looking for answers, I took the pills, but before long I realized that they weren't the answer for me. I could understand the logic: Prozac prevents serotonin, the calming agent we discussed earlier, from being absorbed by the brain. This helps us even out, making us less susceptible to the chemical imbalances that can trigger obsessive behavior. But for me, while there were certainly biochemical issues involved, it was the emotional and psychological factors that I needed help understanding.

Once I realized that this particular therapist was not the right person to help me, I moved on. I eventually met Susi, who ended up being exactly what I needed. I knew from our first conversation that this was going to be different. We didn't talk about how much I weighed or what I was or wasn't eating. Instead, our weekly sessions and phone calls were filled with questions about why I believed I had to be thin, and why I was so sure that everyone else thought about weight the same way I did. By challenging what I believed, Susi helped me recognize some of the lies that had become truth to me. And because I could tell she was genuinely interested in me as a person and respected me in spite of the fact that I didn't have everything figured out, I found myself wanting to work even harder at untangling the web of lies that had ensnared me.

I am thankful now that I was able to recognize and move on from the approaches that did not speak to the core of my problem. My positive experience with Susi has reminded me of the value of finding the right therapist.

The Church

For many who seek the comfort and structure of counsel that is based on spiritual principles, the church is often the first place they turn to when working through personal issues. Indeed, in my own life, those in the church have often served as an important foundation and a tremendous help in times of need, for which I am incredibly thankful. But it is important to be aware of the fact that many times leaders and counselors in the church are not equipped to offer balanced and informed counsel to those struggling with eating disorders. Though their desire to help is genuine, their lack of understanding combined with an oversimplification of the problem can sometimes do more harm than good.

For instance, one of the most damaging statements I've heard is, "If you continue this behavior, you are sinning against God." For those who might not fully understand the mind-set of someone who has an eating disorder, this approach seems fail-safe since most people wish to remain in good standing with God. The flaw in this method of reasoning is that, while our refusal to accept truth may certainly indicate a lack of trust in God, the idea that our behavior is damaging not only to ourselves but also to our standing with God serves only to increase the fear we are already operating out of. And if we simply "stop" our behavior so that we are no longer "sinning," we are left with unresolved issues that are sure to flare up again in a moment of weakness. This is what happened to my mother. The first time she flirted with bulimia, the leadership of the church told her to stop immediately, which she did. But this short-lived episode was only surface evidence of a deeper problem. We both believe that if she had been given healthy counsel at that pivotal moment—balancing spiritual truths with mental, physical, and emotional realities—she might have been spared the intense suffering she faced with disordered eating several years later.

A similarly discouraging response is "If you pray hard enough, God will remove this desire (for thinness) from you." It's not that I don't believe in the power of prayer—in my own fight for freedom from this cage, prayer has played an integral part. But often God has answered those prayers by connecting me with people who offer wise and informed counsel and who help me understand the whys behind my behavior.

The truth is, we are dealing with an issue that affects us on many levels. As we discussed in the previous chapter, sometimes food addictions need to be dealt with. In other cases, the binge-purge cycle needs to be methodically broken. For all who struggle, the issue of self-acceptance, which lies at the core of disordered eating, needs to be addressed. Because of these realities, it's important not to focus exclusively on the role of just one aspect in our recovery. Discounting any part of the equation—emotional, physical, mental, or spiritual—can leave us feeling as if there's no way out.

So What?

Depending on where we are on the eating continuum, good help can be hard to find. But it's out there. Until we find the help we need, we must continue to seek an approach that balances truth with understanding and respect for the person and that addresses all of our issues: emotional, physical, mental, and spiritual.

1. What therapies have you found helpful in your own recovery?

2. What approaches have not been helpful? Why?

3. How do you feel when people misunderstand your disordered eating?

Triggers

Everything was going just fine, until someone commented on the size of my arms.

—LAURA, age twenty-four

I'm ready to get out," I told Susi one day on the phone. I had slowly but surely grown disgusted with living life inside the thin cage, and I felt ready to start making some changes. "That's great," she said, "but it's important for you to realize that there are going to be things that will come up to trigger you back into your old habits."

Susi advised me to make a list of these triggers so that when they occurred I would be prepared to handle them. This section includes many of the things on my list. As you will see, these triggers can be obvious, or more often than not, seemingly innocuous. The important thing is to discover for yourself those situations or events that might trigger your weird eating habits, and then take steps to prepare in advance for how to handle them when they pop up.

Recognizing the Traps

Fashion

Oh, the incredibly exciting world of fashion! The glitzy, glamorous view of how we all should be. I am quite sure I'm not alone in saying that at times we can find ourselves completely consumed with attaining the perfect body as portrayed in fashion magazines. This has certainly been true in my life.

When my clothes didn't fit the way I wanted them to, I would find inspiration to lose more weight by looking at the waiflike images I found in fashion layouts. For many years it was very difficult for me to give up striving for the unattainable images in the media to pursue the appropriate, healthy, and attainable picture of beauty I should seek.

Does the fact that fashion often represents an image that is difficult to attain make it wrong? Not necessarily. I think that fashion, like all art, represents creative expression to be enjoyed by all of us. But it's important to understand that many of the images portrayed in the fashion world can have a harmful effect on those of us who use such examples as a gauge of how we should look. And considering that most fashion models are thinner than 98 percent of American women,[1] the word *model* is actually a bit of a contradiction anyway.

Television

Although the Hollywood community has paid a price for the ultrathin ideal, television programming continues to project images that glorify a barely-there body. Even programs developed by and for the average woman struggle to maintain their relevance in a culture that seems to have a love/hate relationship with excessive weight loss. Tracy White, a former producer for Oprah's Oxygen Network, explains, "The [ultrathin] cycle continues being perpetuated for a variety of reasons.... Because we [the networks] are beholden to Madison Avenue, where the advertising is, the show needs to be a hit."[2]

White goes on to explain that the American public, even those tired of the never-ending drive to lose weight, still can't seem to get enough of thin women on TV. If programs and networks want to stay alive, they must continue to dish out what we clamor for—healthy or not. Some networks like Oxygen strive for as much balance as possible, focusing much of their content on presenting real-world perspectives to their viewers. But in spite of the few programs on TV that do promote a healthy body image, shows projecting an ultrathin ideal continue to be an easy trigger for those of us consumed with attaining the perfect body.

Music Videos and Pop Stars

Like other areas of the entertainment world, the music community plays a cause-and-effect role in the drive for thinness. With the advent of the music video in the eighties, artists gifted at communicating through the intangible beauty of an interesting voice or a well-crafted song were suddenly faced with an intense pressure to develop an equally compelling visual image. Twenty years later the music of today more often places prominence on the "look" of an artist rather than on the relevance of his or her message.

Some recording artists fight the focus on image, and in doing so, they find a large audience thirsty for the message they bring. Whether it's Alanis Morissette celebrating the freedom of self-acceptance,[3] India.Arie soulfully inspiring us to value our uniqueness,[4] or the ever outspoken Pink challenging the shallow nature of the music industry,[5] artists who refuse to be defined by the expectations of the media give voice to the millions of women who long to live free from the pressure to meet unattainable ideals.

But while these celebrated artists have left an indelible mark on our culture, many more have become willing pawns in propagating the airbrushed view of beauty and thinness that now holds them and us captive. For many music fans, this trigger is hard to escape.

The Mall and Clothes Shopping

For a person who struggles to accept herself, an experience as simple as going to the mall can provoke increased feelings of inadequacy and competition. When you consider that the purpose of retail marketing is to remind consumers that there is something they are lacking, it is no wonder that a brief visit can leave us feeling empty and discouraged. It can be difficult to remember that we do not need to achieve the beauty we see in the store windows.

Irregular Eating and Yo-Yo Dieting

Irregular eating patterns can be an added strain to our eating, since each failure triggers us into more eating or further restricting. But I have found that breaking the cycle of yo-yo dieting is not terribly complex. What it takes is a resolve to eat normally for several days—three regular meals or six small meals. After the first two or three days of normal eating, it becomes much easier to fall into a consistent and unfrenzied mind-set and eventually to make this a new eating pattern. In my experience, after even the second day, my stomach would feel better, and I would feel thinner—or at least not fatter. This would help me feel less out of control, which is particularly helpful, since the feeling of being out of control seems to fuel the frustrated eating cycle.

The Gym

The problem with the gym is that we can always find a reason to be un-happy with where we are in the process of getting fit. Anytime we are in an environment focused on image and body shape, we are naturally going to be compelled to continue—and even increase—our unhealthy behavior. That doesn't mean we have to abandon our fitness routine, but it's important to be aware of the possibility that being in a fitness-oriented environment can trigger increased dissatisfaction with our body. We need to prepare ourselves ahead of time so that we can be in a healthy frame of mind when we work out.

Summer and Bathing Suits

Summertime is a huge trigger for most of us. First, there is the gearing-up process during which we lament our winter indulgences and evaluate how much work we will need to do to be ready to bare our bodies for the sake of a tan. Next is the often humiliating experience of buying a new swimsuit, which requires that we must face our bodies in all their dimpled glory under unkind fluorescent lighting. As we examine our reflection, we resolve to take immediate measures to reduce the fat on our thighs and hips. We simply can't accept the "us" that everyone else is going to see.

The trick to conquering this trigger is to take an objective look around next time we're at the beach. Underneath the tans of many women are the same dimpled thighs and soft tummies. Besides, people are often too busy with their own issues to notice the parts of our bodies we despise most.

Friends and Family

Without realizing it, our friends and family members can unintentionally play a part in our obsession. Simple statements or comments about how we look can serve either to trigger a fearful reaction—"You're looking good, like you've gained a little weight"—or to further reinforce our belief that we are on the right path with our unhealthy behavior—"Wow, I wish I looked like you!"

Soon after deciding I wanted out of the cage, I shared some of my struggles with my friend Becky. As I walked her through my experiences, I told her that I felt I was making progress and I knew this would eventually translate into some gained pounds. A few months later Becky said to me, "You're looking better… It's okay for me to say that, right?" "Of course," I replied, but later I had to do some serious reckoning with myself to get over the initial discomfort and fear her statement caused.

There will always be well-meaning friends and family who say innocent things that our warped minds turn into something else. When this happens our only chance for success is to come to grips with who we are and how we're going to address this issue for ourselves. Through my own experiences, I know that this works. And though it's never easy, it does get easier.

School Environments

Recently I received an e-mail from Emily, a freshman in high school. She writes,

> I've been having a harder time with eating since I started going to my new school. Lots of the girls are super thin, and they look at me like I'm just a big pig. I don't want to be one of those girls who's always throwing up, but honestly, I don't know what to do.

Janie, a fourth-grader, tells me, "All my friends are on a diet. It's just not cool to actually eat lunch. We just sit around the [lunch] table and talk instead."

Chelsea, a college junior, writes, "Everyone [on campus] has some kind of eating disorder. I mean really—I don't know anyone who isn't a little concerned about what they weigh. It's hard not to think about it when everyone else is."

For these and so many other students, school environments can be real trigger points for disordered eating. But in spite of the incredible pressure to fit in, it is possible to chart our own course and to find the freedom of choosing to accept our individuality.

Work Environments

While I was still at the record company, I began to realize that working there was a trigger for me. It's not that there was anything inherently wrong with the environment, but being there affected my personality and psyche in unhealthy ways. Due to the nature of the music and entertainment industry, there was a constant focus on image and appearance. Since I was in the marketing department, I could not escape the everyday discussions that reinforced the importance of attractive imaging in order to successfully market our artists. What this translated to in my warped brain was a feeling that I, too, needed to have an image of my own that would stack up against those artists we represented.

I remember talking with Susi about this prior to leaving the company. I admitted to her that one of the reasons I felt so unable to change my thinking patterns was that I was afraid I would let down the people I worked with. I felt that if I was not thin, it would have a negative effect on my relevance as a marketing person. This wouldn't be as much of a struggle for me now, but at that time I was not able to stay healthy in such an environment.

Sugar

As we discussed earlier, sugar intake and overeating cycles are often linked. Most of us know that refined sugars are not good for us. We even avoid giving them to children because we don't want them all wound up. Why then is it hard to remember that sugar can affect adults negatively as well?

You might try this experiment: The next time you are hungry for a snack, try something like pretzels or crackers instead of something sweet. Monitor yourself to see if this food satisfies and calms you. To make the experiment more conclusive, try it once, and then the next time, opt for something sweet. See if you feel different after eating the candy rather than the pretzels or crackers.

Alcohol

If we think that sugar may be a factor in our disordered eating, it can be especially important to avoid alcoholic beverages. Alcohol has such a high concentration of sugar that it has earned the distinction of being "the ultimate refined carbohydrate."[6] For those of us who struggle with an addiction to sugar, just one drink can set off a physiological craving to eat. This craving, combined with the fact that alcohol weakens our resolve, is a sure recipe for disaster.

While alcohol can trigger overeating for the chronic dieter, it often has the opposite effect on many bulimics and chronic bingers. Mom tells me, "It is common for bulimics and binge eaters to use alcohol to help them relax, thus hopefully making them less prone to binge." But this, too, can be problematic. She notes, "It is because of this that alcoholism is common among bulimics and binge eaters."

Wherever we are on the eating continuum, it is important to recognize the potentially damaging effects of this mood-altering substance.

Marijuana

Pigging out seems to go hand in hand with the use of marijuana, as it's commonly understood that smoking pot gives you the munchies. But the real problem can go much deeper. For example, those who are under its influence often feel free of all of their self-imposed rules about what they can or can't eat. Many disordered eaters take advantage of this newfound freedom and binge on all the foods that aren't normally allowed. Once the buzz wears off, the fear sets in and triggers another cycle of dieting to make up for the binge. For those who regularly smoke marijuana, the binge-starve pattern can become a never-ending roller coaster of ups and downs, feast and famine. Resisting the use of marijuana and other illicit drugs will save us much frustration, not to mention the inherent fear, danger, and guilt that accompany any illegal drug use.

The Pill (Oral Contraceptives)

While it may seem obvious that illegal drugs can be problematic, it's important to know that any drug, legal or not, can influence our eating patterns. For example, the pill, one of the most widely prescribed drugs for birth control as well as other medical conditions, often triggers frustrated eating and can intensify already problematic eating behaviors.

I first began to realize the pill was triggering my frustrated eating about a year before I started coming to terms with my disorder. After having been on it for just a year or two, I started to notice a recurring trend. I realized that on the last day of "blank" pills, just before I started back up for the next month, I suddenly wasn't thinking about food. It was just like that! One day I realized, "You know, I haven't thought about food yet today!" This was huge for me, since most of the time I couldn't stop thinking about food and about wanting to eat.

Not long after that I stopped taking the pill altogether. After a short time, I found myself much less consumed with wanting to eat. Of course, my desire to be thinner was still alive and well, but at least I wasn't frustrated and distracted by an urgent desire to be eating all the time. This helped me focus better and kept me from eating more than I needed to.

You may not have the same reaction to the pill as I did, but if you are on the pill, you should still check to see if it might be triggering frustrated eating patterns. The best way to do this is to monitor yourself while you're having your period. If at the end of your period (prior to starting back up on the pill), you realize you are less frustrated about eating, you may want to consult a physician to see whether you should try a different brand or a lower dosage or even discontinue taking the drug until you can get other aspects of your disorder under control. Whatever you decide, it is important that you not make any changes without first consulting your physician.

Your Period

Just as the pill can affect our eating, so can our period—even when we're pill-free. Our menstrual cycle causes a change in our hormones and serotonin levels, thus affecting our emotions, cravings, and of course, making us feel bloated. Bloating is a huge trigger to the eating cycle. Here's how it works:

> You're frustrated because even though you haven't changed your eating, you feel bloated, and your pants are tighter, so…
>
> > You eat out of frustration.
>
> Now you feel like you'd better not eat anymore so you can make up for it, but…
>
> > You're still hungry, so you eat more.
>
> At the end of your period, the bloating has subsided, but you've gained weight as a result of your frustrated eating, and…
>
> > The cycle of frustrated eating continues.

The best thing we can do during our period is to maintain consistency in our intake of food. I'm not talking about strict rules. I'm just saying that we have to make ourselves aware of the pitfalls and talk ourselves through them without giving in to eating more than we should out of frustration. We just have to remind ourselves that our clothes will indeed fit us after a few days of bloating, and though it's hard while we're in the middle of it, we'll be fine once it's over.

Scales

As I mentioned earlier, I believe that, for many of us, scales do more damage than good. However, as I've made my way through some of my struggles, I have found the scale to be helpful for the first time. While I once avoided it entirely, now that I am trying to maintain and even gain weight, I do check the scale from time to time to determine whether I am accurately gauging my weight. In most cases, I'll think I've gained a few pounds only to discover I haven't.

Since our weight can and will fluctuate, many professionals suggest that we should weigh ourselves no more than once a week, and they encourage us to consider the overall trend of our weight rather than fixating on a particular day's number.

When choosing whether to weigh or not to weigh, the important thing for all of us to consider is, "What am I going to do with the information?" If you know that seeing a higher weight will only trigger you to freak out and turn back to weird eating for a few days, then the only healthy choice is to stay away from the scale. But if the information will help you learn how to properly gauge your weight, then go ahead and weigh yourself, but remember: *Use with caution!*

Eating Disorder Stories and Group Therapy

Eating disorders are often unintentionally fueled through products and resources created to help, not harm, a healthy body image. For some people, reading personal accounts of others who struggle only pushes them further into their unhealthy behavior. While these kinds of accounts do offer important insight and perspective that can help people come to grips with their own unhealthy thought patterns and behaviors, they can become problematic for those who are searching for new ways to lose weight.

Another potential trigger can be group therapy. One of my friends tells me how she and her sister would go to group therapy sessions for eating disorders just so they could get new tips on what weight-loss method was working for someone else. They would also go through books, magazines, and Web sites with the same purpose in mind—to further develop their own disorder.

Because of this, I advocate using caution when it comes to participating in group-type therapy for your disordered eating. Unless you already have a desire to come to grips with your disorder—even if that means gaining or maintaining weight—being placed in a room with a bunch of women who all want to lose weight may only trigger your disordered eating further.

Having said that, I should note that many people, both professionals and laypersons, speak of the merits of group therapy. Dr. Donald Durham notes, "Groups offer what individual therapy can't—that is, they increase the sense of universalism, decrease shame, and give the sufferer a sense of empowerment, allowing them to help others while finding help for themselves."[7]

So again we come to an issue of balance. The important thing is to know your motives. If being part of a group session is just an excuse to trigger yourself into continued dieting, then make the choice not to go.

"Buddies"

Cathy stands in the hallway, waiting for Jean to appear. Together they drive to the local Barnes and Noble and head straight for the magazine rack in the back of the store. As they thumb through magazines, soaking in all the latest fashions, they agonize together over how they'll never measure up.

"Look," says Cathy. "Her arms are *so* small! Maybe if I just cut back a little I can have arms like that too."

"Yeah," agrees Jean. "I mean, if she was able to get that thin, there must be something we could do too."

Later that afternoon Cathy and Jean are at the library, surfing the Internet to find the "proanorexia" sites. "I don't want to be anorexic," says Cathy. "I just want to see if there are any quick tips on how to lose a little weight."

Lindsay and Maggie have a different kind of buddy relationship. They both choose to ignore the other's blatant weird-eating habits. Together they split a small bowl of fruit and a diet soda and call it lunch. They talk about which foods have fewer calories and how you can eat more of this type of potato chip because it has no fat. But they never admit that they might have issues with food.

While many who suffer with weight obsession tend to close out most of the people around them, for some of us, there is this interesting little phenomenon called the buddy system. After all, misery loves company. And even though those of us who are caught in the trap often don't recognize our own unhappiness, we know that it's easier to stick with the program when we are around others who seem driven toward the same goal.

This is important to consider as we begin to reach a point where we long to look beyond the bars of our cage. Once we've decided we want out, it's important that we begin eliminating daily social interaction with people who might trigger our disordered thinking.

Along the same lines, we need to seek out friends who we believe have a healthy self-image and try to spend more time with them. In my own recovery, I found that surrounding myself with people who I knew weren't focused on how thin I was (or wasn't) made it easier for me to place less priority on my weight as well.

Stress

Stress triggers disordered eating even for those who have no issues with weight. For those who do, its influence can be especially hard to avoid. When we feel stress, we tend to eat or not eat depending on our personality. Stress also impairs our ability to be reasonable, as everything seems to take on a heightened sense of importance. Sometimes it's necessary to stop in the middle of a stressful situation and remind ourselves that this too shall pass. It is also important to have a healthy outlet for stress, such as exercising, being creative, or spending time with friends. Stress can't rule our lives if we are prepared to handle it when it comes.

Events and Special Occasions

Like most women, I am affected by events, especially those that involve a lot of people I may not have seen in a while. Most of us want to be more beautiful and, yes, thinner than the last time others saw us. So it is common to try to lose weight for an upcoming wedding, a high-school reunion, or other such occasions. As I've made progress in my recovery, I've noticed that though I still struggle with these thoughts, I can honestly say I worry much less than before. Earlier in my disorder I would starve myself for days, sometimes weeks, to make sure that I looked thin and attractive at an event. Now I just try to make sure I look decent, and I have to tell you, it's quite a relief not to have to always be thinner and thinner.

The important thing to realize is that people probably won't notice if we're a few pounds heavier (or lighter) at the reunion. If we can just accept this, maybe we can all enjoy life a little more.

So What?

The triggers that shake us are different for every person. It's important to know that they do exist and that they don't need to have power over us. Being aware of what our triggers are is the first step in overcoming the hold they have on us.

My Triggers

1. What things seem to trigger an unhealthy response in you when it comes to weight and eating. Write down as many as you can think of here. (To help stimulate your thinking, you might want to review the triggers mentioned in this chapter.)

The Message of the Tapes

I've already eaten breakfast, but a chocolate-covered doughnut is being offered to me. I don't need the doughnut, but I *want* the doughnut. It's small, about a quarter the size of a full-size doughnut. It really wouldn't count if I ate it anyway because I'm in a work meeting. Jane had three and she's bigger than I am, so I should be able to eat one. Stephanie is sitting next to me, and she's not eating the doughnuts. She's cute and thin. She'll think I'm fat and gross if I eat it in front of her. She probably thinks this about me just because I have it on a plate and will be eating it. I'll eat the doughnut when she walks away.

Yuck! That doughnut tastes like wax. It's bad. I won't "miss" anything if I don't eat the rest of it. Why should I waste calories on something that bad? But I've already taken a bite. I can't throw it away…there are starving children in this world. If I eat it fast, then it won't count.

I just ruined the day. I started out so well with a balanced, healthy breakfast. I couldn't resist the doughnut. I might as well eat fat unhealthy foods for the rest of the day. My pants are tighter. My stomach is sticking out further than it was before I ate the doughnut. Maybe if I drink twenty-four ounces of water it'll dilute the bad contents of the doughnut, and I can flush it out of my system before it does too much damage. I've failed… I can't even decline the offer of a doughnut.

It's clogging my arteries right now.

—JESSIE, age thirty-four, on eating a chocolate doughnut

T hink you're the only one who struggles with an incessant voice in your head that tells you you're never going to measure up? Just like Jessie, for those of us who place an unhealthy focus on our weight, normally inconsequential events build up to catastrophic proportions in our minds and soon become "tapes" that we can't escape.

Nonstop Chatter

Inspired by the imagery of the "Message of the Arrows" that authors John Eldredge and Brent Curtis paint in their thought-provoking book *The Sacred Romance,* I realized one day that the most constant and destructive force in my battle for a positive self-image was the "message of the tapes." These tapes represent an ongoing internal dialogue that spurs on our unhealthy behaviors. Messages such as, *I'm not as thin as she is… If I eat that I'll gain weight… These pants seem tighter today than last time I wore them… They don't love me because I'm not thin.*

At every turn, at each event, and with every new pair of jeans, I was confronted by the tapes. Soon I had become so used to them that I didn't even realize they were there. To be honest, even if I had realized what was going on, I probably wouldn't have wanted the tapes to be silenced for fear I'd take advantage of my newfound freedom and head to the nearest McDonald's.

It wasn't until I decided to get help with my obsession that I recognized how pervasive the tapes had become. As I started to consider breaking out of the cage, the volume of the messages seemed only to increase.

As I tried to explain this to a friend of mine, I said, "It's as if every minute of every day is spent thinking about food, being thin, feeling fat. It's like a never-ending tape in my brain." She didn't get it. She couldn't understand how this could absolutely consume me, especially since I carried on a demanding yet seemingly normal life. And even if I was a little obsessed, everyone wants to be thin, so who cared if I thought about it all the time? What my friend couldn't appreciate was how dramatically my life had been affected by these thoughts. She didn't know how dangerous listening to these tapes can be.

Sound Bites

So what do the tapes sound like? A friend of mine recently shared hers with me:

> If you eat this, everyone will think you're a pig.
>
> If you eat this, you are childish and unhealthy.
>
> If you eat this, you will show weakness.
>
> If you eat this, you will cancel out any exercise you've done this week.
>
> If you eat this, you have no self-control.
>
> If you get fat, you will not be respected at work.
>
> If you get fat, you won't have any physical beauty.
>
> If you eat this, people will think, *No wonder she's overweight.*
>
> If you eat this, you will disappoint God.
>
> If you eat this, God won't love you as much.
>
> If you eat this, God and everyone at the table will know what a bad person you are.
>
> If you eat this, people will think you're ignorant.
>
> If you eat this, you won't be special because of your size.
>
> If you eat this, you will have to pay for it for the rest of the week by not eating breakfast or lunch.
>
> If your clothes fit too tightly, it means you are a horrible person who should have known better than to eat too much.
>
> If you eat dessert, you may as well give up on having any self-control ever again.
>
> If you start to get fat, you will not be able to stop. You will lose control.
>
> Any unhealthy food is like poison in your system that you will never get rid of.

Wow! Such incessant self-badgering might be expected of one who is mentally insane, but this particular woman is very bright and quite talented. She holds down a demanding full-time job and is happily married. Yet she suffers from fears, habits, and feelings of failure that no one would guess she struggles with.

"Jessie," who shared the chocolate doughnut story, adds these messages from her own personal tapes:

> If I eat this, my clothes will instantly be tighter.
>
> If I lift weights or exercise, I will instantly look more toned.
>
> I can't say no to someone who's offering me food.
>
> I have to eat the whole thing.
>
> If I drink a lot of water, it'll "displace" the effects of what I've eaten.
>
> If I eat it fast, it won't count.
>
> Goal: Wake up with a hollow empty feeling in my stomach.
>
> It is good if my stomach is growling before a meal.
>
> My identity is in how much I weigh.
>
> If I eat this, I will be comforted.
>
> I'm going to eat that because I deserve it.
>
> If she can eat it, I can eat it.
>
> If I eat that, I'll look fat.
>
> If I don't eat it now, there won't be any left.
>
> I'm a failure when I overeat.
>
> Eating relieves stress.
>
> Eating gives me something to do.
>
> I have to eat at 7:00, 12:00, and 6:00 because that's what I've always done—whether I'm hungry or not.

Like both of these women, millions of us have developed our own personalized tapes of rules and regulations. Daily we live enslaved to the accusing voice that plays over and over in our minds, relentlessly repeating the same strains, invariably rewinding to the part about how fat we are. These tapes have become such an integral part of us that we can't imagine being free from them. But freedom is out there.

Turning Down the Volume

The tapes can't just be turned off as an instant benefit of deciding to deal with our disordered eating, but they can gradually lose their strength. It's now been a couple of years since I told my friend about my tapes. I'm post-first-weight-gain-in-ten-years, post-obsessing-about-food-every-minute-of-every-day, and life is different. It really is. I still struggle sometimes, but I can honestly say that the tapes are no longer playing. Once in a while I hear a little "commercial," a brief ten-seconder: *Are you sure you don't want to lose a little weight? Wouldn't you rather skip that high-fat meal?* But through practice—and by the grace of God—I'm able to switch off the sound and get on with my day.

For me it took a process of small steps, but the volume of the messages continued to decrease, until one day I realized that I had not thought about food, weight, thinness, or fatness for hours. It was a glorious moment.

So What?

Turning off the never-ending negative tapes gives us the ability to reclaim our productive, creative, and sensitive minds. What things we can accomplish when we're not consumed with the negative!

What's Your Tape Playing?

1. List the messages about food, eating, and weight that play in your mind. Try to write down as many specifics as you can. Put a check by those that seem to be the most pervasive.

2. In any given hour, what percentage of your thoughts are consumed with these tapes?

3. What would you think about if the tapes were suddenly turned off?

Prayer

God, give me the courage to admit to myself that my ideas about eating and weight have begun to control how I live my life.

Give me wisdom to understand what might trigger my feelings of fear and insecurity, and bring someone into my path who I can talk to about my struggles.

In times of discouragement, help me believe that who I am is more important than what I weigh.

I want to live free from the negative voices.

PART 4

A GOOD DOSE OF THE TRUTH

One of the hardest parts of working through disordered eating and poor body image is realizing how distorted the truth has become in our minds. We have been conditioned to believe untruths such as "If I'm not thin, they won't love me" or "If I could only lose ten pounds, everything would be better" to the point that lies often seem to outnumber truths in our lives. Unfortunately, when we live in a world of false-isms, we lose sight of right and wrong, and the stabilizing power of true reality disappears.

A friend of mine recently underwent a double mastectomy to remove the beginning traces of the breast cancer that had touched nearly every woman in her family. One day I asked her about this, trying to understand how she possibly could have gone through such a traumatic event and is now living a seemingly normal life. As we talked I admitted to her that I was not that comfortable doing breast self-exams, probably because I was afraid of what I'd find (the truth).

"That's ridiculous," she exclaimed. "Breast cancer does not always have to be the end of the world. Sure, there's a period of truly horrible stuff, and things happen that you never imagined you would have to deal with emotionally, physically, and mentally, but then it's over. Life can go on."

Wow. I had never heard anyone talk this way about cancer. In my mind, it was always the biggest, scariest thing you could face because it meant life was over. But for my friend, finding that little pea-size lump was truth, and knowing the truth allowed her to do something about it. For her, seeking the truth was a step toward freedom.

In this section, we'll take a step back and reevaluate the role that truth—and lies—have played in our obsession with weight. The goal is to arm ourselves with truth and to learn how to lean on that truth to find our own freedom.

Our Excuses and the Price We Pay

Nothing is easier than self-deceit. For what a man wishes, that he also believes to be true.

—DEMOSTHENES, 384–322 B.C.

My daughter won't get fat. I'm always going to be there to make sure she eats right. It's my responsibility as a mother to make sure she doesn't have to go through the terror I faced as a fat kid.

—HALEIGH, age thirty

Most of us have a host of arguments ready to throw out to anyone who suggests we focus on eating better. We've considered them carefully and are quite convinced of their logic. But for every excuse we choose to live by, there is a truth that we have chosen to ignore—and a price we've never considered.

Flawed Logic

It wasn't until I started meeting with Susi that I began to question the logic behind some of my excuses for my disordered eating. In the weeks and months that followed my first counseling session, I continued to be surprised at how many lies I had taken for truth. Following are just a few of the many excuses that Susi challenged.

"I Am Happy with Where I Am"

Because I considered thinness to be my greatest achievement, for many years I genuinely believed that I was happy living within the strict parameters of my disorder. At the time I didn't regret not being able to eat a normal meal or the fact that some women seemed anxious to avoid a relationship with me. I truly believed I was content with my life. This is why it was so pivotal for me to acknowledge that there was a lot I was *not* happy about. For so long I had everything I thought I wanted, but once I began to think objectively, I realized that in many ways my life was unrewarding and frustrating. It was this knowledge that led me further into desiring freedom from the cage I knew I was in.

"My Health Is Not Being Affected"

As I've mentioned earlier, for many years I received a clean bill of health from my doctor, which convinced me that I was getting by on very few calories with little or no impact on my body. But I was wrong. As I entered my late twenties, I began to realize that I was chronically fatigued. My immune system also seemed to be breaking down, and I started to develop allergies for the first time. For several years my intestines were particularly sensitive to certain foods, and urinary tract infections became a fact of life. More than anything, I could never seem to feel good.

Dr. Gregory Jantz, author of *Hope, Help, and Healing for Eating Disorders,* explains: "It's possible to seem outwardly healthy… Even your bloodwork is going to stay there for a while, but there comes a breaking point."[1] Indeed, as we grow older, we are likely to begin seeing the effects of our lack of nutrition. Some problems may seem minor, while others can have more devastating consequences.

In 2002 pop music sensation Anastacia told VH1 that her efforts to lose weight to meet the music industry ideal had landed her in the hospital. With regret she says, "I tried to be smaller and I did lose a lot of weight, but I didn't realize what it would do to my intestines." As a result of her disordered eating, Anastacia was diagnosed with Crohn's disease, a serious chronic inflammation of the gastrointestinal tract. She has now returned to a healthy view of her body, saying, "I'd rather be a chunky singer than a really unhealthy girl who keeps on seeing herself in a light that doesn't fit."[2]

Unhealthy eating can have serious effects on the reproductive system as well. While many disordered eaters are able to experience healthy pregnancies, chronic dieting and disordered eating have been linked to infertility. Australian researcher J. X. Wang tells us, "Being underweight or overweight has an adverse effect on reproduction."[3] Dr. C. Wayne Callaway, a weight specialist at George Washington University Hospital in Washington, D.C., echoes this concern, warning his patients who diet and/or exercise excessively that they will have difficulty becoming pregnant.[4]

Even if we have a strong constitution and our body seems to hold up under the strain of our unhealthy eating practices, our mental and emotional capacities still suffer from a lack of nutrition to the brain. Our bodies were created for a balanced intake of nutrients. It is illogical to believe that we can achieve optimum health while starving ourselves.

"I Have This Thing Totally Under Control"

Many of us see our eating as something we can control. After all, *no one* can make us eat something we don't want to. *We* choose what we want to weigh. *We* are the strong, the mighty, the disciplined. Or are we?

I remember vividly the day I first realized that I was not in control of my disorder. We had just moved into our first home, and I went out to mow our tiny lawn. As a young girl, I had found solace in working outside, and after years of apartment life, I was excited to have a little patch of grass of my own.

I was barely finished with the front lawn when suddenly I felt as if I might pass out. For the first time I got angry. In that moment, I realized that I had sacrificed my health and well-being for way too long, as even normal tasks now required more effort than they should. I could not believe that this thing I thought I was in control of was actually in control of me!

For so many of us, being able to control our diet gives the illusion that we are in control. More often than not, however, if we consider the rules we've come to live by, we would see that we're not really the controlling party. It is our fear of fat, motivated by our need for acceptance, that is controlling our lives to the extent that just eating a snack requires creative reasoning and bargaining with our captor.

"I Don't Have Time to Learn a Different Way to Eat"

Before I left my full-time job, I couldn't have imagined adjusting my busy life to allow time for learning a new approach to food and eating. I was so wrapped up in what I considered to be my "important" life that it seemed incredibly difficult to switch gears.

It didn't take long for me to discover that eating normally was actually easier than chronic dieting. Being able to order anything I wanted off the menu opened up a whole new selection of restaurants when I was in a hurry for lunch. Shopping for groceries became easier when I learned that I had many more choices available now that my criteria were not incredibly specific. One of my friends told me that she can spend ten minutes shopping for just one item as she methodically reads each label to determine which product fits her restrictive diet. Truly, this must be more draining than learning to eat without fear. Even if it does take some time to relearn proper eating habits, the payoff is well worth the investment.

Read the Fine Print: Hidden Costs Apply

Even as I began to come to terms with the truth behind my own excuses, it took some time for me to believe that there were compelling reasons to change my eating habits and attitudes toward weight. I knew I was not technically sick, and I liked the attention that having a thin body gained me. From a practical standpoint, it was less expensive to eat out, clothes always hung just right on my body, and I never needed to take a break from my busy job to eat lunch—not to mention the fact that most everyone praised me for my thinness. With all of these benefits, I had a hard time seeing the downside of my obsession. In fact, it was only as I began to examine my life closely that the hidden costs started adding up.

Time

As we've discussed, those of us who place an unhealthy focus on weight control tend to think about food constantly. It was only as I started breaking free of the message of the tapes that I began to see how much of my time and energy had gone into maintaining my weight. I then began to realize that all the time I spent thinking about my body and my weight, trying to lose a pound or two, and hoping that no one would notice I had eaten an off-limits food item could have been much better spent on something productive. Also, since starving myself caused me to be constantly fatigued, I wasted many evenings and weekends lying in bed, barely finding the energy to keep my house clean, much less to go out and exercise the creative and recreational parts of my brain. My constant inner battle drained me of all my energy and left little room for social relationships that could have helped boost my self-confidence and overall sense of well-being. I soon came to realize that time was one of the most unfortunate sacrifices I had made during the many years I had been consumed with being thin.

Quality of Life

It is difficult to lead an enriched life when we spend every waking moment warring against ourselves. I often sacrificed the quality of my life in favor of protecting my obsession. For example, in addition to going into starvation mode before any social event, I would skip out on events that might jeopardize my well-controlled eating plan. There were many times my diet-induced fatigue kept me from doing things I would have enjoyed, but it took me years to realize the price I had paid.

Now that I am no longer consumed with eating and weight, I have found that I have more time and energy to develop and maintain meaningful relationships. Because I am not worried about what others will think of me, it is easier to make friends, especially with other women. And while my life used to revolve around my job and my diet, it is now packed full of interesting challenges, enjoyable activities, and rewarding relationships. Looking back, it shocks and saddens me to think that I willingly gave away more than a decade of living well.

Joy

Have you ever noticed that many women who diet, even those who are successful at it, don't seem particularly joyful? At first glance they may appear to be happy, but a closer look often reveals a troubled look in their eyes.

The truth is, we often sacrifice joy when we obsess about our weight. Even at my thinnest, I was no more joyful than when I was carrying around the extra pounds I gained in college. It's paradoxical because we've been taught that being thin will bring us happiness, but when we are at war with our bodies, true joy is elusive. Only when we understand that we are worthy of love regardless of what we weigh will we find real joy.

New Opportunities

When we allow ourselves to believe that we have to be thin to be accepted, we often miss out on opportunities that might be just what we need to find excitement and creativity in our lives. Similarly, it is difficult to develop our gifts and talents when all our efforts are focused on eating, dieting, and controlling our weight.

Probably the most rewarding things I've found as I've begun to break out of the cage are the freedom and confidence to pursue old dreams and new challenges. Since I am no longer bound by a need for the approval of others, I feel empowered to pursue my dreams in a way that was never before possible.

Relationships

Recently a man told me how much his girlfriend's obsession with her weight has tested their relationship. Because she struggles with accepting her body, she continually rejects his romantic gestures, rebutting each endearment with "How could you say I'm pretty? You know I'm just a fat pig!" It is difficult for him to understand why she won't accept that he loves her as she is, curves and all. "When she says these things, it just sucks the life out of the room," he told me.

Another friend of mine constantly complains to her husband that her thighs have somehow grown larger overnight. After many failed attempts at dissuading her from her ridiculous claims, her husband often has to leave the house, frustrated that no matter what he says, his wife refuses to believe him.

It is undeniable that our self-loathing can damage a loving relationship. How ironic it is that even when those we love confirm that our obsessions are unhealthy, we simply refuse to see the truth. After a while, it becomes nearly impossible for us to believe anything but the lies we've built up around us.

Peace

"Nothing fairer than peace is given to man to know; / Better one peace than countless triumphs," noted early Roman poet Silius Italicus.[5] Indeed, the peace that eludes us when we strive to meet unrealistic expectations is ours to gain when we accept ourselves as we are. There is nothing like the peace of knowing that our value does not rest on how we look or what we weigh.

Security

During the height of my controlling behavior, when my body fit the strictest standards projected by the media, I felt every bit as insecure as I did during the days of unwanted weight gain in college. Even though I was happier with the way my body looked, my need for others to notice and approve of me seemed much more pronounced during this time. I was also afraid that if I gained weight, everyone would lose respect for me. It took me awhile to understand that when our measure of self-worth depends on the number on the scale or on the size we wear, our very security becomes linked to something that is inherently insecure.

Money

While many of the costs of disordered eating are paid in intangible currencies, there is a significant financial expense that should be considered as well.

For instance, during my college binging phases, I would gladly plunk down my hard-earned cash in exchange for large amounts of food. Following each binge, which could be quite expensive on its own, I would frantically purchase diet products such as Slim-Fast, water pills, or even laxatives to "make up" for the weight I had gained. During this frustrating period, I was willing to spend whatever it took to get my weight back under control.

As the binges came to an end and I headed into chronic dieting, the financial impact of my disordered eating seemed less obvious. After all, I could go out to eat and order a small dinner salad instead of a big meal. And since I ate only one meal a day at some points, my grocery bill was significantly lower than what my friends seemed to spend. But while I was spending less money on food, I was spending more on the clothes, makeup, and hair that now seemed essential in maintaining the image I had become obsessed with projecting. While there was nothing wrong with my desire to look good, I had slowly but surely become a slave to improving my appearance, whatever the price.

According to Margo Maine in her book *Body Wars,* Americans spend more than 50 billion dollars each year on dieting and diet-related products.[6] Fifty BILLION! If you're like me, that number is probably beyond comprehension, so let me put it into context for you: A person would have to spend a million dollars a day for just under 136 years to go through that amount of money.

On a more practical level, just consider how much we're willing to spend on diet programs, metabolism boosters, fat blockers, exercise machines, meal replacement shakes, specially formulated prepackaged foods, and even plastic surgery. Even if we're able to avoid these more obvious expenditures, the cost of name-brand low-fat products can significantly increase the grocery bill, with such products averaging around 40 percent more per ounce than their nondiet counterparts. And when we add in the cost of therapy, prescription drugs, or in some cases, hospitalization, disordered eating can hit the wallet especially hard.

Imagine how different things would be if our dollars went to things we really enjoy, those things that rejuvenate our soul and make us thrilled with living.

The Greatest Cost of All: Propagating the Cycle

As we consider the hidden costs associated with our obsession, it is important to understand the greatest price of all: By choosing to believe that thinness is more valuable than our mental, physical, and emotional health, we become willing participants in propagating the very thinking that has caged us. And while the damage we do to our peers is undeniable, it pales in comparison to the curse we are passing along to the most innocent victims in the game: our children.

Our Legacy

"God knew *not* to give me a daughter," writes Sarah, a thirty-five-year-old mother of two who has struggled with disordered eating for most of her adult life. As heartbreaking as her statement is, Sarah is the rare person who recognizes the damaging effects that her unhealthy views on eating could have on her children. For many of us, our fear of fat causes us to start taking precautionary measures early to ensure that our child does not grow up heavy.

As a new mother, I have experienced this danger firsthand. When I thought my one-year-old son was gaining weight too quickly, I decided to "help" things by switching him from whole milk to a lower-fat variety. Following a firm reprimand from his pediatrician, I was forced to recognize that my fears had led me to do something that could potentially have harmed my son. Even though I know deep inside that it is perfectly healthy and normal for my son to be a chubby baby, there are still days when I worry that his passion for food might turn into a weight problem. In times like these, I have to remind myself to back off and let his body adjust to its own natural growth pattern. I also have to admit to myself that weight might still be more of an issue for me than I'd like it to be.

As our children develop, they are increasingly able to sense our discomfort with weight, whether our own or theirs. Even if weight never becomes an issue for them during childhood, our behavior often leaves a lasting impression that can evidence itself later in their lives. I was recently reminded of this during a conversation with my mother when she revealed that her mom (my grandmother) had frequently made statements about her own "fat stomach" when my mom was a young girl. As an impressionable child who wished to live up to her mother's expectations, my mom began to fixate on her own growing body, particularly her belly. To this day, my mom still regards her belly with disdain, even though she is not overweight.

Saving Them from the Pain

We often hear stories of parents who impose diets on their children to "save them from the pain of being fat"—like the milk incident with my son. While this can seem like a worthy cause, we often overlook the painful lack of self-confidence we instill in our children by teaching them that only certain body types are acceptable.

In September 2002 psychologist, author, and talk-show host Dr. Phil dedicated an entire show to the problem of eating disorders and obesity among children. Wisely, he took issue with the parents, not the children. When one mother explained that she had pushed her daughter to lose weight because she wanted to spare her the pain of societal rejection, Dr. Phil challenged her, saying that such pain would "pale in comparison to the fact that she [her daughter] never had the love and acceptance from her mother that was the foundation from which she built everything else in her life."[7]

As I watched this mother continue to make her case, it was easy to appreciate her logic. Much of her argument was based on culturally accepted theory—*thin* people get better jobs, overweight women *never* appear in commercials—but she was missing the point many of us fail to see: One of the best gifts we can give our children is the knowledge that what they weigh does not have to dictate their value as a person or their enjoyment of life.

My friend Jeannie has been an inspiration to me on this front. One day early in my progress she shared with me the story of how she had come to terms with her own disordered eating and attitudes about weight for the sake of her children. Her first motivation was the obvious—she needed to allow herself to eat properly to ensure a healthy pregnancy. When her children became teenagers, she continued to resist the urge to fall back into old patterns, realizing that if she allowed herself once again to restrict her diet, her example could adversely influence her children, particularly her oldest daughter who was just beginning to deal with the to-be-expected body-image woes that accompany adolescence.

Jeannie still struggles with feeling fat, but she is determined to spare her daughters the pain and frustration that go along with the self-defeating practices of an eating disorder. And while she has a hard time accepting the few pounds she still wishes she could lose, she makes every effort to avoid voicing her frustrations, choosing instead to reinforce to her daughters that "being curvy is just fine."

When Jeannie first told me her story, I was still fairly entrenched in my fear of fat, and I couldn't help but think, "If it was *my* daughter, I would want her to try to be thin because that is definitely preferable to being heavy." But Jeannie had the wisdom to know that her daughter would only suffer if she became a slave to the thin ideal that simply wasn't her body type.

Now, as a mother, I can finally appreciate the selfless wisdom that Jeannie has chosen to live by. Honestly, I am still a little nervous about how well I will handle the issue of weight if and when it comes up with my son or any future children. But I know that regardless of what society says, it is far more valuable for our children to have a healthy body image and enjoy life free from the cage of our expectations than for them to try to fit the image of beauty projected by our culture. I will arm myself with this truth daily as I face the many challenges of being a parent.

So What?

We must take the brave step of admitting that our excuses for unhealthy behavior are probably flawed. Nothing comes without a price. Often the cost seems reasonable, since what we want never seems as expensive as what we need. But in the end, we will most certainly sacrifice something of lasting value in our efforts to attain the elusive and empty prize of perfection.

1. Take a few moments to write down your most common responses when someone expresses concern about your eating habits and/or weight. After you have done so, place a check mark next to those responses that you can objectively say are not true.

2. Which of the hidden costs, if any, mentioned in this chapter do you feel
    you have paid as a result of your unhealthy views on weight and eating?

3. How does it make you feel to know that your views on weight might
    inspire others, including your children, to diet?

4. What does your response to the previous question tell you about your own
    fears?

Sex Appeal Does Not Equal True Acceptance

If I gain weight, men won't think I'm attractive anymore, and then where will I be?

—Susan, a forty-two-year-old single mom

One all-important indication that a woman has the culturally correct body image is the attention she gets from men.

—Sharlene Hesse-Biber, *Am I Thin Enough Yet?*

As we discussed earlier, our culture's unhealthy focus on sex appeal often plays into our issues with eating and weight. Because this subject is too often skipped over, especially in more conservative circles, I feel compelled to address it here, even though doing so requires me to shine a light on yet another unattractive scene in my own personal story.

Throughout the ages sex has been glorified as the one undeniable power a woman holds. While some have raised their voices against the sexist views of women, many women continue to believe that if they can only be thin *and* sexy, they will find the happiness that eludes them. I know that in my own fight for approval, the power of sexual attraction was a weapon I wielded forcefully. With this tool I could obtain what I most desired—money, influence, social status, and the biggest prize, the acceptance of men. But what I didn't realize was that I was walking into another trap.

The Sex-Equals-Power Trap

After graduating from Bible college at the age of nineteen, I spent about three years in Dallas exploring the world on my own terms. I took a job as a waitress in a busy downtown restaurant and, for the first time, was immersed in an environment that was fully approving of casual sex.

Like many girls growing up in the seventies and eighties, I had been sexually aware from a fairly young age, but my Christian upbringing had taught me the value of waiting until marriage to have sex. It wasn't until I was surrounded by people who had such liberal views on sex that I began to learn about the so-called power of my sexuality.

Initially, I was a little frightened of the men who now surrounded me, many of whom had very different ideas than I did about life, love, and God. And with the ever-present threat of AIDS that was paramount in the early nineties, the stakes seemed very high. But in spite of these concerns, it wasn't long before I found myself crossing the proverbial line.

At first, I became codependently attached to the men I was involved with. I would get incredibly jealous if they looked at other women, and I always felt insecure about whether they were going to stick around. But one day, weary of the constant emotional drain, I came to the conclusion that if I could just turn off my feelings, I could become the rejecter instead of the rejected. That day I made a decision: Men were no longer going to have control over me. So for a few years I moved from one relationship to another, many of which I didn't even enjoy, but I reveled in knowing that I was the one calling the shots.

In the early days of this period, I was curiously flippant about my lifestyle, noting in my journal, "I feel strangely unbothered by it all…" But it wasn't long before I recognized the emptiness of my pursuits. This entry appears just a few months after the previous one:

> I'm lonely. I've come to realize I care more deeply about things than I
> thought I did. Now I'm feeling hurt… I can't keep my feelings shut off
> forever. I must be true to myself… Constance, feel! Allow yourself to
> feel again…

It turns out that Sex Equals Power was just another trap. The bait was "Be sexy and you will have whatever you desire." But the truth was, my efforts to gain the acceptance of men only made me less able to accept myself as I was. The trap said, "You are the one in charge," but the truth was that I often felt out of control, telling my journal time and again, "I didn't really want to do it, but I felt like I should," or even, "I hate myself for doing this."

Not surprisingly, it was during this period of time that I entered my most stringent phase of chronic dieting. I was trapped in what seemed to be a self-perpetuating cycle: I wanted to be thin so that more men would find me sexually attractive, and feeling more sexually attractive boosted my incentive to keep dieting. This cycle continued for several years, robbing me of the joy of healthy relationships and skewing my perspective of myself and my body.

Thankfully, this period ended when I met my husband at the age of twenty-two. In AJ's arms I found reciprocal love and acceptance, and when we decided to get married, I thought the games were over—I was wrong.

Lingering Dangers

Recently a woman named Tina contacted me to discuss a "really tough time" she was going through. Her e-mails leading up to our conversation spoke of "feeling guilty…doing things I don't want to do," phrases that sounded strangely familiar. I began to wonder if she was talking about more than just her unhealthy dieting practices. When we finally talked on the phone, I learned that she had fallen into an inappropriate relationship with a man she had recently met. "It's hard," she said. "I love my husband so much, and he's the most important thing to me, but I've grown so attached to the attention I'm getting from this other man. It's filling a need for me right now that my husband just can't seem to meet."

Alarm bells sounded off in my brain. I knew where this was headed—I'd been there before. I, too, had played Russian roulette in the early days of my marriage, deceiving myself about what was right and what was unequivocally wrong. Like Tina, I knew I had been blessed with the amazing gift of my husband, and yet I found myself hungry for something more. Even though I couldn't imagine living without AJ, I still struggled with a need for acceptance. Instead of realizing that I needed to learn to how to accept myself, I continued to seek out the approving glances of other men, which had made me feel so accepted in the past. This often had the potential to lead me into dangerous territory.

As Tina continued her story, I knew of only one response. "Break it off," I implored. "*Now.*" As I know only too well, when it comes to defending a marriage—which even in the most difficult of situations is an investment worth protecting—the voice of reason must shout loudly from the rooftops, "Be not deceived. This will truly end in death... Death of a relationship. Death of love. Death of your spirit. No good can come of this. *End it now!*"

Thankfully, this same voice of reason had pushed me to run from my flirtations before they got to a point of no return. As my husband stood by me, broken yet lovingly resolute, I was shaken to realize that I had almost traded in my gold for dirty, lifeless ashes that had masqueraded as the answer to all my problems.

Several years later, as I began to work through these issues with Susi, it became apparent that I still believed the lie that true acceptance and sexual attraction were the same thing. Even though I was determined to avoid any opportunity for an improper relationship, I had continued to assume that my sexuality was what made me special, and in my mind, thinness was essential for that sexuality.

Breaking Free

I can honestly say that I no longer place such value in the power of seduction. I have learned that while our culture celebrates sex appeal as the key to finding the fulfillment we desire, its promises are false. Indeed, in the context of a loving, monogamous relationship, sex is beautiful, intoxicating, comforting, and secure. But outside that context, its luster is lost. We may still experience momentary feelings of pleasure and satisfaction, but in their wake come feelings of confusion, frustration, insecurity, fear, and emptiness.

Even if we think we've successfully turned off our natural inclination to become emotionally attached, it is against our nature to stay numb forever. As author Wendy Shalit points out, "If being blasé about sex were natural, why would so many women have to be on Prozac in order to carry out what their culture expects of them?"[1] Only by returning to the modesty that guided us as innocent children can we rediscover our true selves…and find the love that will sustain us.

Sex Appeal and the Single Person

I realize that for single women who long to be married, all this talk of monogamy may seem a distant hope and the need for sex appeal more important. While attraction is certainly a key element when it comes to finding a mate, believing that sex appeal will somehow gain you true acceptance will only keep you from finding the love you seek.

I can see that if I had not put so much focus on my sexuality when I was single, I would have been spared the many relationships that only numbed my sensitivities and clouded my view of what was important.

When I met my husband, attraction was definitely part of our relationship, but I quickly came to understand that what he was really interested in had little to do with how my body looked. It is a deeper love that has sustained us through eight years of marriage so far, some of them very difficult. This same love continues to make our relationship stronger with each passing year.

The key here is that all of us deserve to be loved by someone who is interested in us for more than just our physical appearance. But we can't expect to find that person when we're working our hardest to prove that we can play the sex-appeal game. The best relationships are those that require no games and allow for the joy of discovering one another in a safe and secure relationship. Choosing to make decisions without giving in to our culture's demand for sex appeal is often the first step toward ending the games.

So What?

While sex appeal plays an important role in the human experience, it does not bring us any closer to finding true contentment. Learning to see the beauty in the nonsexual aspects of who we are will allow us to reclaim our true self, not the self we think is expected of us.

1. How has a desire to be sexy factored into your obsession with being thin?

2. Have you found yourself risking your health, relationships, or well-being for the sake of the approval of men? In what ways?

3. List some things about yourself that you think are attractive, apart from outward sex appeal.

Chapter 20

It's All About Perspective

Beauty is as relative as light and dark...

—PAUL KLEE (1879–1940)

When I was young, I thought thirty was old. Now forty sounds young.

—CINDI, forty-seven-year-old wife and mother

One of the ironies of living with disordered eating is that we not only believe the truth is a lie, but we take subjective ideas as absolute truths. For example, beauty, size, and even importance can mean different things to different people. It all depends on our perspective.

Beauty

I was recently reminded of the subjective nature of beauty when talking with my friend Rachel, who is rather tall. One evening she told me that she had always hated her height and wished she could be shorter. Describing herself as "all arms and legs," she explained that she often felt awkward and unattractive because of how tall she was. As we talked, she commented on a mutual friend of ours who was shorter and more petite. "I would feel more attractive and feminine if I was like Jill," she said.

I was surprised by her statement. I knew that Jill had always wished she were taller and had even taken to wearing shoes with very high heels to simulate the effect. To Rachel, being tall was a curse, but from Jill's perspective, it was just the opposite.

The truth is, when it comes to real beauty, there are no absolutes. What is beautiful to one person may be ugly in the eyes of another, and vice versa. When we focus on meeting a rigid and unrealistic standard of what it means to be beautiful, we can't appreciate the beauty of our own uniqueness.

On Makeup

While we're on the subject of beauty, let's talk for a moment about makeup. While younger girls these days seem to place less importance on this age-old ritual, those of us born in the seventies or earlier probably feel quite attached to the concept of "putting on" our faces before we leave the house.

One day a few months back, I was talking with my neighbor Julie. I commented during our conversation how I really loved my house but wished we had a bigger lot. (The houses in our neighborhood are jammed closely together.) I explained to her how I hated having to see my neighbors every time I went to the mailbox. She nodded sympathetically. I continued, "I mean, what if I don't have my makeup on?" At this she looked at me quizzically, "Oh, I never worry about that." Suddenly something clicked in my brain. If *she* doesn't care about wearing makeup, then she probably doesn't care if *I* wear makeup. So Julie became the first person I visited regularly without worrying about applying makeup beforehand. I mean, she's just across the street. How ridiculous is it for me to get all gussied up to impress this person who doesn't care anyway? If she doesn't care, why should I?

After this initial revelation, I became bolder about leaving the house without being "properly" made up. With each plain-faced trek to the grocery store, post office, or even to Starbucks, I realized that I was less and less concerned about what everyone else thought of the way I looked. The truth is, the more I've gotten used to seeing my face washed clean, the more I realize that there really isn't anything wrong with the way it looks without makeup. And while I can appreciate that I probably do look more attractive with some cosmetic help, I can now accept who I am without it, even in public.

Makeup can be a great way to improve our appearance, and it's important to feel good about how we look, but I think it's very freeing to realize that who we are under the makeup is okay. In the same way, who we are inside our body is okay too. It's understanding that we are not what we weigh or what we wear or what we have that makes us special. It's who we are beneath the painted mask.

Fat

A friend of mine who is often a guest speaker for women's events tells of the day she had lunch with three other women, all of whom were new moms. Over lunch the topic of discussion turned to complaints about all the weight these women had put on during their pregnancies. At the peak of the discussion, one of them exclaimed, "And can you believe, I actually weighed [x] at full term?!" The other women all nodded supportively, while my friend's mouth dropped open. The weight this woman was so upset about was my friend's target weight at Weight Watchers!

Of course, when my friend tells this story, she immediately wins fans in the audience. It seems that we often need to be reminded that fat is a subjective term. In some cultures, weighing more is desirable because it speaks of wealth and station in life. Yet in our postmodern American culture, the natural curviness of a woman's figure is often considered fat and is looked down upon.

When obsessing about the weight we wish we could lose, it's helpful to remember that what is fat to one person is often a goal for someone else. And fat is not just about numbers on a scale. A woman who weighs 150 pounds and has a proportioned body can actually appear to be slimmer than someone who weighs 15 pounds less and has a different body shape. So depending upon our perspective, fat can mean different things to different people.

Thin

Thin is just as subjective a term as *fat*. In fact, the thinner we get, the less thin we often feel. Except in cases of obesity where it is not uncommon for people to believe that they are thinner than they really are, most of us believe that when we put on weight, we definitely are getting heavier. So why is it that when we're taking it off, it never seems to be enough?

In doing research for this book, I came across some "pro-ana" Web sites that feature startling and tragic images of anorexia, and I can honestly say I have never wanted to look like that. My heart breaks to see the power of the lie that can make us believe we should starve ourselves to the point of death.

But I have always had an ideal of thinness in my mind. It has changed over the years, depending on how healthy and balanced my view was at the time. As a young girl with no reason to worry, I liked my slender size 6 or 7 body. In the midst of my chronic dieting, I felt that I should be no larger than a 2. At that time I would have been horrified to fit into a 6—a size that some women dream of. I can now understand—and believe—that more weight actually looks better on me, and so my definition of thin is changing as I move into a healthier place. But even as I'm making peace with a larger allowance for "thin", there will probably always be someone who will look at me and find a few pounds they think I should lose.

"Important"

One night I was trying to locate a friend who I had gone to college with more than ten years ago. A new record label I was doing some consulting for was seeking some "unsigned" artists, and Shannon immediately came to mind. A dynamic vocalist, pianist, and songwriter, Shannon had an extraordinary gift that few are blessed with. So I got on the Internet and looked her up. As I clicked my way through the search engines, I began to realize that this girl had been quite busy since college. Not only had she been involved with several recordings, but she had become a clinician for a workshop that attracted musicians from all over the world.

As I went through these sites, I came across other names I knew from my days in college. Several of the people I had toured with as a teen in choir were now key vocalists, musicians, songwriters, and worship leaders at large events and churches.

I have to admit, it took a little wind out of my sails to see this. I had to confess to myself that I had become rather bigheaded about all the things I thought I was accomplishing. It's funny how we can become incredibly proud even in well-doing. Part of this stems from the fact that we seem to hang our self-worth on the hanger of our accomplishments. Even with the truest of intentions, it's hard not to begin feeling self-important as our dreams begin to take shape.

But *important* is a subjective term. Just when I was considering myself and all the things I was doing to be important, I was brought back to earth by looking beyond the small circle of my immediate surroundings.

For many of us, *thin* equals *important.* But when we understand that *important* is itself a subjective term, we are left to question what our endless pursuit of thinness is truly gaining us.

Recognizing Reality—Really!

One of the results of living in a subjective world is that it is easy to have an unrealistic picture of ourselves—which often means assuming the worst about ourselves. Too often we focus so intently on our flaws that we lose touch with the good things that others see in us.

Recently I was on a tour bus traveling to Texas with a company I had done some consulting work for. On our last night, coming back to Nashville, several of us fell into an interesting discussion, prompted by one of the women asking me about the book I was working on.

Five of us women sitting in the front section of this very comfortable tour bus started talking about how we focus a lot of our time on image, eating, and weight. Though each of us had a different story, we were inescapably connected by the commonalities we share as women.

Across from me sat Misty, an outgoing, intelligent twenty-something who had become a who's who at the different schools she had attended. An average size 10/12, Misty has an admittedly straight build as opposed to a more hourglass figure.

Next to Misty was Heidi, a statuesque, fuller-figured woman. Each of us had remarked to each other during the trip how beautiful we thought she was. This girl had it all—long, luxurious dark hair, a sexy figure, a strikingly pretty face, and a commanding presence.

Sitting to my left was AnnJanette. Another twenty-something, AnnJanette was also quite curvy, and though she didn't fit the cultural standards of ultrathin, she was quite attractive, whether dressed up or wearing jeans and a T-shirt. Add to that her beautiful brown hair, full mouth, and great skin, and she really could turn a few heads.

Also sitting to my left was Marlei, a woman coming up on forty who looked more like thirty with her pixie face and cute figure. She has never struggled with issues of eating and weight, and her body has always been naturally slender.

As we started to talk about the so-called thin cage, it was fascinating to hear each of these women share things that I would never have guessed prior to our conversation.

After Marlei, who had always been more focused on intelligence than beauty, Misty seemed to have the healthiest body image of us all. Somehow at a young age, she had made peace with the fact that her body did not meet the tall-and-thin ideal. While she definitely kept an eye on her weight, she was not at all consumed with worrying that she was not thin enough. In fact, she sees her flaws as a blessing because they afford her instant friendship with most of the women she meets rather than inviting the intimidated glares we as women so often fire in the direction of anyone we consider more beautiful than ourselves. She explained to us that one day she finally understood that we are here to be "vessels of love" for one another. Not in a creepy, weird way, but because we, especially as women, have a gift of loving one another. When we are so caught up in the game of appearances, we are not able to fully experience and share this gift.

I stared, incredulous, as she went on to explain that she had learned early in life that she was not defined by how she looked. Little did she know that this concept was the basis for my own recovery and the foundation for this book!

Heidi sat beside her, soaking all this in, and then she suddenly got the nerve to speak. "I don't know if I should admit this," she said and then went on to tell us how she was consumed with worrying that she was not thin enough. Apparently she had gained twenty pounds over the course of nine years of marriage and was feeling rather unattractive.

I was dumbfounded. You would think that since I always have this topic on the brain, I would have seen this one coming, but I didn't. "Wow," I told her. "I've spent this whole trip thinking you are a great example of a woman who is really a woman and how attractive that is!" She was quite surprised by my statement. Then, one by one, the other girls chimed in, each echoing my appraisal of Heidi and her beauty.

It was apparent that Heidi was as taken aback by our admiration as we were by her admission of frustration.

And then Marlei made an incredible point: "The problem is that what you've been focusing on is not reality," she told Heidi. "What we've just shared here is actual reality."

Reality Is....

Marlei's statement was another "aha" moment for me. So many of us spend all of our energy listening to the false messages of the tapes going on in our head, even though those tapes are based on the subjective truths of our world instead of on real truths. If we could live in reality mode, we'd understand that we are fine just as we are, without all the abuse we inflict on ourselves daily.

Here are some truths to hold on to. Reality is:

• You don't have to be pencil-thin to be loved.

• You are probably not as fat as you think you are.

• Even if you are not incredibly thin, there are probably others who could only dream of weighing what you do.

• Becoming something you were never meant (built) to be will not bring you happiness.

• We are drawn to those who seem to know who they are and are content with themselves.

• Being thinner is not going to make you better at your job.

• Many guys appreciate a woman's natural curves.

• Your value is not determined by how thin you are.

• Wearing a smaller size is not going to change who you are.

Of course, there will always be realities that seem to combat the truths that give us hope. For example, it is reality that:

- we live in a society that judges women harshly on appearance;
- some of the people who love you might think you look better when you've lost a little weight;
- the fat girl gets picked on in school;
- there are not very many curvy women in the media these days.

Yes, these things—and many others—are true. But we have the choice to seek positive or negative reality in our lives. While we can't escape from the realities we wish weren't there, we *can* focus more of our time on the realities that resonate in our soul, telling us that we are valid just as we are and giving us hope to take the next step toward loving ourselves.

This concept has been freeing to me. Since gaining weight during my pregnancy, I've often gone back to my husband—probably at least once a week—for a reality check. "Are you sure I look better now that I've gained weight?" AJ always assures me that I look so much better now that I'm getting more nutrition in my body: "You'd look great even if you gained a few more pounds." I can now see that he's right. This is the reality I choose to accept. I know that it's true, and I choose to listen to that truth instead of the lie that says, "You were more interesting when you were thinner."

Seeing with New Eyes

When I was thinner, I would get all decked out for an event and stride in with my head held high, assuming that everyone thought I was incredibly attractive and fascinating and successful because I had achieved such remarkable thinness.

The reality—though I didn't know it at the time—was that what others saw was an insecure and unhealthy girl who felt she had something to prove. Those who loved me worried about my health. Those trapped in the same cage I was in retreated even further into their shells, vowing to emerge triumphantly thinner than I at our next encounter. Those who knew me casually probably didn't care either way.

What was truth? What was real? Now, stepping back from it all, I can see the whole picture with new eyes. The reality is that I was not a complete person when I was so consumed with being the thinnest girl in the room. Recognizing this reality has been an important step for me in reclaiming my right to live life to the fullest.

So What?

When we consider that we live in a subjective world, especially when it comes to appearances, we are free to reclaim our uniqueness. Assured in the confidence that beauty (and thinness) means something different to everyone, we can allow ourselves to widen our perspective and embrace true reality.

1. How does it make you feel to consider that not everyone has the same ideas you do about what is attractive, thin, or important?

2. Look at the messages of the tapes you listed in chapter 17. Which of your messages reflect reality and which don't? (If you're not sure, ask someone who genuinely cares about you to offer his or her opinion.)

3. Do you want to live in reality or fiction? Why?

Chapter 21

On Getting Older

When I was in my thirties, I had these little square hips left over from being pregnant, and I just hated it. I kept thinking, "All those years before, I had a perfect glamour-girl body, and I didn't spend one minute appreciating it because I thought my nose had a bump in it." And now that I'm old, my shoulder hurts and I don't sleep good and my knuckles swell up, and I think, "All those years in my thirties and forties I had a body where everything worked perfect. And I didn't spend one minute appreciating it because I thought I had square hips."

—ALICE GREER, from *Pigs in Heaven* by Barbara Kingsolver

To know how to grow old is the master-work of wisdom and one of the most difficult chapters in the great art of living.

—HENRI AMIEL, 1874

I've spent a fair amount of time in this book discussing our culture's mandate that thin equals beautiful, but I would be remiss to ignore another powerful cultural message: thin equals youthful. For teens and college students reading this book, this might not be a factor yet, but for many women, the root of our obsession with dieting is the fear of getting older.

Indeed, for those of us no longer in our twenties, staying thin seems to be our only option when it comes to preventing the appearance of aging. As the wrinkles set in, we tell ourselves that if we can just lose a few more pounds, no one will notice that we're getting older.

The cruel irony is that chronic dieting and unhealthy eating practices can actually cause us to age prematurely as we routinely deprive our bodies of the nutrients, vitamins, and rest required to achieve optimum health and vibrancy. But we pay little attention to this fact, proud to be able to fit into Junior and Young Miss sizes. After all, being thin makes us feel young, and you're only as old as you feel, right?

The fact is, we're all getting older. None of us will spend our entire lifetime svelte and gorgeous, no matter how many body lifts or botox injections we get!

Unless we learn to accept, even embrace, our aging bodies, we will be at war with ourselves until the day we die.

"But I Fit into This When I Was Sixteen..."

After I first gained weight as a freshman in college, I was crushed to realize that I no longer fit into some of the clothes I had worn in high school. A couple of years after that initial weight gain, I came across a very slim white denim skirt in the back of my closet. As I held it up against my larger body, I despairingly thought to myself, *This is impossible! How am I ever going to fit into this again?* From that day on, fitting into that skirt became a fixation for me. I was afraid, and unwilling, to accept that I no longer had my teenage body.

Now, twelve years later, I am a woman in my thirties. Add to that the fact that my hips, pelvis, and abdomen were stretched nearly to bursting during pregnancy and the delivery of my son, and it's understandable that I might not be able to fit into the clothes I wore when I was a girl. I have had to come to a place of peace with this fact.

I have also had to accept that the skin on my neck is no longer smooth and supple. I've had to swallow the jagged little pill that my breasts, after months of nursing, are never again going to look the way they once did. And I've had to deal with knowing that my profile—particularly under the chin—no longer has a strong edge to it, something that causes me no small measure of frustration. But the important thing is that I'm making peace with these things.

Whether it's being able to share clothes with our daughters or to fit into our wedding dress again, many of us fixate on clothing size as a measure of our youthfulness. All this focus on fighting the natural process of aging robs us of the joy we find when we can embrace the women we are becoming.

Learning to Embrace Aging

Why have we decided that growing older is something to be avoided at all costs? If we stop to consider what we really believe about aging, we most likely will discover that our feelings on the subject are curiously mixed. For example, when seeking wise counsel, we are often drawn to those older than ourselves, knowing that they have valuable life experiences from which to offer us meaningful advice. And when we look into the eyes of our parents and grandparents, we have no trouble seeing the beauty that lies beneath the laugh lines and sunspots. Yet we are so unforgiving with ourselves. Too often we spend our days mourning and fighting the passing of our youth. Because we feel that each step away from our twenties and thirties is another step toward becoming obsolete, we war against ourselves, intent on preserving and manipulating our bodies to retain the youth that falsely promises acceptance. In wrestling with our bodies, we sacrifice cultivating and enriching our souls—the part of us that will outlast everything else.

"I Need to Look Young to Attract a Mate"

As more women are marrying in their thirties and forties, whether for the first time or following a divorce or the death of a spouse, the added pressure of attracting a mate can fuel our fear of aging. As my friend Inger says, "I can't help but think about how I look. Until I find a husband, I've got to keep in shape, because there's a lot of competition out there."

Although this is an understandable concern, it must be balanced against the truth that when Mr. Right finally does come along, he has to love you for more than your body if your relationship is going to work. And not all guys are seeking a superslim mate. I see many women who have no trouble attracting men even though they are not a petite size 4 or 6. In fact, it seems that the older we get, the more forgiving we become of each other's shortcomings. We must remind ourselves that just as we are able and willing to love someone for more than just physical appearance, we are also worthy of that same love.

The fact is, all of us can choose to embrace and enjoy the person we are now, or we can waste each day in what Sydney Smith would call, "That sign of old age, extolling the past at the expense of the present."[1] Unfortunately, many of us choose the latter. In our efforts to avoid the inevitable, we miss out on discovering who we really are beyond our external appearance. Then one day we wake up, startled to discover that our body has betrayed even our most dedicated efforts at preserving our youth, as the mirror presents to us a person we hardly recognize.

The Stranger in the Mirror

A few years ago a friend of mine in her midforties explained to me her frustration with the fact that, although she felt no different than when she was twenty-nine, when she looked in the mirror, a stranger seemed to be staring back at her. As a young and invincible twenty-six-year-old, I'd never heard this expressed before, and I must admit it concerned me. The idea of arriving at the midlife point and hating my reflection was, and still is, a little scary, to say the least.

I've come to realize that how we handle our aging bodies depends on our definition of beauty. If we are seeking external beauty—rock-hard thighs, a full mouth, pregravity-affected skin—then yes, it is fleeting. But if we can look beyond the surface to find the beauty that lies deep within each of us, then we can rest in the knowledge that true beauty never dies...it only grows richer as it matures.

Those of us who choose to believe that we must remain externally youthful and beautiful in order to be worth the space we take up will never learn to make peace with the stranger in the mirror. With each passing year, we will only grow more frustrated with ourselves, stunting and even killing our inner spirit as we continually reject our reflected self.

If Only

Like it or not, we are all growing older, and the natural process of aging seems to dictate that our bodies will change with each passing year. And while it is certainly appropriate to make efforts to maintain a healthy lifestyle, including proper nutrition and exercise, we must also place priority on developing our inner person so that when our body does begin to break down, we will have something deeper and more meaningful with which to sustain ourselves.

As we enter what are supposed to be our golden years, we will worry more about the generation that follows us than whether our swimsuit shows our sagging butt. Our most rewarding moments will be visits from our children and grandchildren rather than the joy of fitting into that elusive size 4 or 2.

When we near the end of our life, we won't be thinking, "If only I had achieved a thinner body." We'll think, "If only I had worried less about the temporary and the unchangeable and spent more time investing in the eternal."

So What?

Aging is an unavoidable fact of life. The earlier we can learn the art of embracing this reality, the more time and energy we will be able to invest in the richness of our future.

1. Has a fear of aging influenced the way you feel about your weight? Explain.

2. What is it about getting older that scares you most? Why?

3. What do you hope to be remembered for after you die?

That Which Defines Us Controls Us

The body is a consuming project…because it provides an important means of self-definition, a way to visibly announce who you are to the world.

—Joan Jacobs Brumburg, *The Body Project*

One day after months of counseling with Susi, I finally dug deep enough to catch a glimpse of the root of my obsession. Buried beneath the tangle of lies was a central core that sustained my unhealthy behavior: I thought that being thin defined who I was. Suddenly the phrase "That which defines us controls us" entered my brain—and changed my life.

As I pondered the implication of this truth, I realized that believing I must be thin to be loved had severely limited my choices when it came to how I lived my life. Because I had placed an inordinate amount of importance on thinness, I couldn't risk losing it. And so what I had looked to as my self-definition had ultimately taken control of my life.

As humans, we naturally seek to define ourselves by the things we think we can control, such as our career, our looks, or the things we own. The problem is that when we allow external things to define us, instead of looking to who we are on the inside, we actually give away our freedom and liberty, because those externals end up controlling us.

For example, a person who is defined by achievement gives up recreation, time with family, and spiritual and interpersonal growth in order to gain success. A person who is defined by her spouse, family, or friends gives up the continued exploration and understanding of herself, choosing instead to be molded into what others want or expect her to be.

Similarly, those of us who are defined by our appearance and weight have become slaves to the rituals of pursuing perfection. And while weight loss in and of itself is not wrong, when we believe that *how thin* we are defines *who* we are, we unwittingly sacrifice the enrichment of our true selves to pursue a definer that falsely promises love and acceptance.

Our True Defining Force

If that which defines us will ultimately end up controlling us, to what can we look for our self-definition without sacrificing our happiness, health, and well-being? Only by allowing ourselves to be defined by who we are on the inside can we be freed from the control of unforgiving definers.

In ancient biblical times, the prophet Samuel was seeking a man to anoint as the next king of Israel. When he found someone he considered a worthy candidate, God challenged him, saying, "Don't look at how handsome Eliab is or how tall he is.... God does not see the same way people see. People look at the outside of a person, but the LORD looks at the heart."[1]

Given this new directive, Samuel passed over his first choice and six others, eventually anointing a youth named David, the smallest and youngest of the candidates. No one could have known then that this unlikely choice would soon become one of the greatest figures in ancient history—a majestic king, a talented musician, and the author of hundreds of psalms, which are still quoted today. The key thing to note is that when choosing David, God looked first at his heart. The rest was of less concern to him.

I believe that God did not intend for us to link our weight to our value. He created each of us uniquely and separately, and we are not supposed to fit into just one standard of weight or body type. And while God sees our struggles and the measures to which we're willing to go to perfect our outside appearance, who we are on the inside is much more important to him than what we look like.

The challenge with finding freedom in this truth is that most of us have a hard time feeling that God's acceptance is enough. Too often it is the approval of others that we so desperately seek, and yet such approval is fleeting at best.

By learning to replace our external definers with the eternal truth that God loves us as we are, we can find the confidence to release ourselves from the hold of the expectations of others. And once we are free, we can begin living richer and more rewarding lives, inspiring those around us to join in the quest for what really matters.

Many Impress, Few Inspire

I was driving to a friend's house the other day, and for some reason I began thinking about a man I had come in contact with during my days in the music business. This guy was in a powerful position and fully enjoyed its benefits. As is often the case, he had also allowed himself to believe in the power of his own importance to the extent that he often forgot about the little guy farther down the ladder. As I quickly moved to judge him, I suddenly realized this could describe several of us working in the music business at that time, myself included. We had decided, whether consciously or otherwise, that our positions made us important. With our flashy titles, we sought to impress everyone we came into contact with. And most of the time we were successful—at least within the small circle of our industry.

Along the same lines, I sought to impress others with my thinness. I felt that being thin sent the message that I was in control, and this feeling of control made me feel powerful. But I was so consumed with maintaining the impressive facade that I rarely took time to develop my character and so had little with which to inspire those around me.

The truth is, many impress, but few inspire. The trouble with seeking to impress is that it requires so little of our heart and soul. But to inspire…that must be the greatest of accomplishments, for inspiring others allows us to be a part of something so much bigger than ourselves.

Recently a friend of mine in her seventies greatly inspired me when she told me that the most important thing she could do was give her life away. Denny's simple statement gave me something to aim for, a goal worthy of pursuit.

Another friend was such an inspiration to me and many others that when he died unexpectedly as the result of a tragic accident, the church could barely contain the thousands who mourned his passing. At his funeral, many spoke openly about how they had been affected by Grant's lust for life and his passion for serving others. Most incredible to me was that even in death, Grant inspired us to live more thoughtfully, passionately, and spiritually minded—an incredible legacy for his wife and young sons.

One of the most inspiring people I've had the privilege to know is my mother's husband, Bud. Ever since the tragic accident that took my mother from an active and energetic lifestyle to a life as a quadriplegic confined to a wheelchair, Bud has ceaselessly worked to handle her personal care and to ensure her comfort wherever possible. An active-duty colonel in the U.S. Air Force and a part-time flight instructor, he has sacrificially adjusted his life to be available to my mother at every turn. All hours of the night he is there by her side in case she wakes up, needing another blanket or sometimes fewer blankets. (Her internal thermostat has been significantly affected by her injury.) I'll save you all the heartbreaking details the caretaker of a quadriplegic must deal with, but suffice it to say, I have seen no greater example of "'til death do us part" in action. Bud remains a constant and present inspiration not only to me but to anyone who has the opportunity to see this love in action.

When considering the big picture of life, it's important that we ask ourselves, "Do I want to seek to impress or live to inspire?" How we answer that question will define how we live. If we seek to impress, then we will continue to feel empty despite each new accomplishment. The increasing importance we place upon our material possessions, appearance, and successes will only serve to bind us up further and further. But when we refuse to be defined by external things, our focus changes, and we are free to inspire others, because we know that our value is in who we are, not how we look.

So What?

When we allow external things to define who we are, we give away our freedom and liberty. By understanding the truth that who we are on the inside is more important than what we look like, we can turn our energy toward loving and inspiring those around us.

What Is Defining You?

1. Take a moment to consider what thing(s) in your life have become definers. In addition to your concerns about weight, what are some other things that seem to have a hold on your happiness? Fill in the blank:

    "Without my _____, I would not be important/worthwhile/special in this world."

    Popular Definers
    - Possessions: *cars, home, clothes, jewelry*
    - Appearance: *thinness, beauty, health and fitness*
    - Achievement: *job, status, success*
    - Relationships: *friends, family, business associates, social clubs and activities*
    - Talents: *music, cooking, gardening, art, acting*
    - What others think of us: *attention, admiration, respect*

2. What is hardest about looking to God's view of you as your definer? Why?

3. How has a desire to impress others influenced your lifestyle?

4. What characteristics about yourself might inspire others?

A Richer Life Awaits Us

When I woke up this morning, I already could tell that changes were happening. I enjoyed my breakfast without worrying about eating too much.
When I picked out what to wear, I picked out what *I* wanted to wear and
not what I thought other people might think I look good in. I am already
sensing that freedom in my spirit. And this is just the right time for this
to be happening—right before the New Year!

—BEATRICE, enjoying her first tastes of freedom

As we close this section, I wish to leave you with the most hopeful truth that is
ours to claim: A richer life awaits us on the other side of our all-consuming
obsession. When we choose to break free from the cage we are in, the happiness
we will find far outweighs the perceived benefits of our unhealthy lifestyle.

Recently my friend Christine asked me how my life was different now that
I'm no longer consumed with dieting. This got me thinking about all the
changes that have occurred since I've been able to see myself as more than just a
"body." I suppose one of the primary differences is that I am not so consumed
with always having to look perfect. But there are many more positive changes,
as I discovered when I began listing them in black and white. Following are just
a few:

- I'm able to eat foods that I loved as a child but as an adult decided were
  off-limits.
- I'm able to sleep.
- My husband likes my slightly curvier body.
- I'm a lot more even-tempered.

- I have a much easier time making friends.
- I don't avoid social situations out of fear that I'll eat something off-limits.
- Clothes look better on me now that there is more "meat" to help fill them out.
- My body seems to maintain a healthy weight on its own.
- My skin looks better and has more color.
- I feel free! I can't really put a finger on that exactly, but the feeling is constant. I don't feel bound up with obsessive thought patterns centering on food and thinness.
- I don't worry that people will not like me if I'm not thin.
- I have so much more "brain time" now for being creative.
- I am learning to see others for who they are, not what they look like.

It can be overwhelming to look at this list and consider that, for many years, I lived with the absence of these things—and probably many others I'm just not thinking of right now.

Life Outside the Cage

Following the enlightening experience of writing my list, I created a section on my Web site (www.findingbalance.com) that asks visitors, "How would your life be different if you didn't struggle with eating and dieting?"

The many responses we've received in just a short time have only proved that, indeed, a much richer life awaits us on the other side of our obsessions. The following lists represent just a few of the responses that have been posted to the site:

Cherie
- I might actually be able to find out who I am.
- I could walk into a room and not have to worry about what other people are thinking of me.
- I could be a much better person, mother, wife, daughter.
- Life would not be so draining.

- I could finally feel free from the prison I've lived in for more than fourteen years.
- I could have a better sexual relationship with my husband.
- I would not be so sad and depressed all the time.
- I could like myself.
- I could have a positive outlook on life and not feel so negative all the time.
- I could feel like I am worthy of love [and] acceptance regardless of how I look.

Kathi

- I would be happier.
- There would be no worrying about how fat I look.
- I wouldn't have to weigh myself every five seconds.
- I would be more active with my friends.
- I wouldn't have to think about the calories and fat in food.
- I wouldn't worry about what can and cannot pass my lips.
- Life would be carefree and simple.
- I wouldn't have to be so secretive.
- I could understand things better.
- I could get through a day without crying myself to sleep at night because of the weight I thought I gained that day.

Lita

- I would not have to wear a jacket with certain outfits to hide my fat.
- I would not want to throw up if I ate too much.
- I could go out and have fun without being so self-conscious.
- I could eat desserts without feeling guilty.
- I would like myself more.
- I would wear sexier clothes.
- I wouldn't have to be so perfect in everything else.
- I would not hate the mirror.

• I would not mind exercising in public.

• I would not eat in secret.

Entry after entry I've received chronicles the I-would-bes of those who realize they're trapped in the cage. Most entries reflect the positives of finding freedom, but some women admitted there are some negatives to changing their behavior. Consider the following entry:

Anonymous Submission
    • I would have a great deal less stress.
    • I would be able to enjoy social situations more without worrying about avoiding food I can't say no to.
    • I would be more easygoing.
    • *I would be fat.*
    • I would not look like I am tired all the time.
    • I would be happier, at least to the extent of eating.
    • *I would be mad at myself for being weak and giving up.*

When I first received this entry, I was a little surprised to see the negative comments mixed in with all the positive differences the writer suggested. But it made me realize an important point: It is healthy and necessary to consider *all* the ways in which our lives might change if we give up this obsession. This writer articulated the very real fears she faces when thinking about changing her behavior. Now she is able to view her fears in the context of her desires and can choose to find a balance between the two.

Talking Back to Our Culture

You may find yourself arguing, "But those things on my list aren't as important as being thin." Our culture's expectations are so strong that it's hard to choose what brings us true joy. I think one key to finding truths we can live with is to step outside what we perceive to be the expectations of our culture and recognize what really makes us happy.

My list of things that make me happy includes:

- Reading a book.
- Taking a nap.
- Eating pizza.
- Hanging out with my husband.
- Playing with my son.
- Taking a long evening walk in the warm summer breeze.

None of these activities involves dieting or trying to be thin, and yet they bring me true joy and contentment.

Now, let's consider what our culture might say about my list:

Reading: "Watch the movie instead; it's faster and more visually stimulating."

Napping: "Why sleep when there is so much you can be doing, like going to the mall, working in the yard, taking your son to the zoo? Besides, lying down slows your metabolism and causes weight gain."

Eating pizza: "Too fattening. Why not have a grilled chicken sandwich instead?"

Hanging out with my husband: "That's okay, but isn't that taking time away from more important things such as writing or cleaning the house?"

Playing with my son: "Yeah, I guess this is a good one. Just make sure you're getting everything else done too."

Taking a long evening walk: "Great, but be sure to pick up the pace. That way you can burn the calories you ate for dinner. And make sure you've got your cutest exercise outfit on in case you run into someone you know."

If I were to plan my day according to the messages of our culture, I would rise early, eat a bagel with fat-free cream cheese for breakfast, go running, come home and work in the garden, make a low-calorie lunch (or a smoothie), run to the mall to pick up a new pair of shoes, see a movie, and then come home and watch television until I fall asleep without even giving my husband so much as a good-night kiss. This is entirely culturally acceptable. But is it acceptable to me? This is the question I must answer if I am to live freely.

The Choice Is Ours

One day my friend Dale made an interesting suggestion: "Why don't you just gain five pounds and see how you feel?" he asked. "Since you know you can take it back off, what do you have to lose?" As I turned his words over in my mind, I found there was something incredibly freeing about this concept. For so long my avoidance of food had been about proving that I could be as thin as I chose to be. Now my friend was suggesting that a choice to gain was just as valid as a choice to lose. He wasn't suggesting that I relinquish control; he was merely suggesting I use my well-developed control for something positive instead of something self-defeating.

The choice was mine. I could choose to accept myself with a little more weight. I could choose to believe that it wasn't the size of my clothes that made me important. I could choose to reclaim my right to my own body. Hmmm… interesting.

For many of us, all that stands in the way of living a richer life is the fear that the self-control we've worked so diligently to cultivate must now be thrown out the window as we meekly give up our will so that we can be considered recovered. But in many ways, making the choice to accept ourselves at any weight only reinforces the power of our own free will.

Consider the words of Terri, a woman in her midforties, who says, "I finally realized this past year that I can either choose to watch what I eat and deny myself all the time and be a size 7, or I can eat what I want, when I want it, and be happy and a size larger. To me, it's worth it to be one size bigger to enjoy my life."

Like Terri, when we grant ourselves permission to choose, we are empowered with the realization that we don't have to stay in bondage to something that is sapping life from us. Choosing freedom is the greatest choice we can make!

So What?

In choosing to accept ourselves without condition, we have the opportunity to reclaim a richly rewarding life. The happiness found in doing so far outweighs the perceived benefits of our unhealthy lifestyle.

1. Take a few moments to consider how your life might be different if you were not consumed with the pursuit of being thin. (Think about both positive and negative changes you might experience.) List as many as you can think of. If you need more space, pull out a sheet of paper and insert it here.

2. If you could step outside the demands of our culture, what types of activities would bring you the most joy?

3. Review your answers to the previous two questions. Do you see how choosing to make peace with the natural size of your body can be so much more rewarding than choosing to live life according to the messages our culture sends? Explain.

Prayer

*God, help me to arm myself with truth
so that I am better equipped to make the choices
that will bring me a fuller, richer life.*

*I realize that in my fear I have chosen to believe many lies,
and I pray that you will continue to expose these lies to me so that
I may walk away from their influence in my life.*

Thank you for giving me a free will and loving me just the way I am.

PART 5

GETTING OUT

Here we are at the end of the road—a moment of choice. I've told my story and pleaded my case, earnestly attempting to paint an honest and balanced picture of the truth about this cage we've been living in. As you've read through this book, you've probably come to some of your own conclusions about what freedom might look like in your own life. Now it's time to consider taking some active steps toward finding that freedom.

These last few chapters are practical bite-size ideas that have been helpful to me as I've broken free from my own thin cage. Following each chapter are questions and action steps to help you start your own process of getting out of the cage.

You may want to look at one step each day or one a week. Or it may be helpful to read through the whole section and then commit to doing one or more of the steps first and the others later. Any approach you choose is fine. The important thing is that you continue to move forward, placing more and more distance between you and your captor. May you find the freedom that is yours to claim.

Starting Simple

It is always the simple that produces the marvelous.

—Amelia E. Barr

Once we've decided to venture out of the cage, we must try not to pressure ourselves to immediately change everything we've come to believe about eating and weight. When considering such a significant life change, we need to give ourselves permission to take our time. Only through a healthy, balanced process will we be able to successfully and completely break free from the lifestyle that has held us captive. This does not mean it is okay to ignore truth under the guise of taking our time, for I believe that once we know truth, we become accountable for what we choose to do with it. But we should afford ourselves the opportunity to take baby steps.

Willing to Be Willing

My own recovery started with a simple prayer: "God, make me willing to be willing." It was my way of saying, "I'm not yet ready to change, but I want to be." What a simple place to begin. My mother recently told me that this had been her own approach as well. There is comfort in knowing that we can start simply and that we don't have to jump to the next stage before we're ready.

Once you pray this prayer, be looking for things to start happening. In my own journey, God showed me that I was not alone by bringing me into contact with Susi, who turned out to be the first person to work with me in a way that was truly helpful. Other things soon followed, including encouraging phone calls from friends, conversations that sparked thought, and newfound dreams that helped nurture the desire in my heart to be free.

It's important to know that we don't have to be in an incredible spiritual place to take this first step. At the time that I began seeking freedom, I was pretty far from God. I did not pray a lot, and I wasn't going to church regularly. But I knew God knew my heart, and it was my heart that I was asking him to change, which he did. I believe God will work with whatever we give him. We don't have to have it all together to begin the process.

Seeking the Art of Being

As we allow our hearts to become more willing to accept truth, an important first goal is what I like to call "seeking the art of being."

The idea here is that before we *do* anything, we must first consider what it means to *be* who we are. For if we can learn to accept who we are as human *beings,* not human *doings,* then our focus will change from achieving a certain weight to learning how to find beauty in who we are on the inside. Once this is the attitude of our heart, everything becomes much easier.

Grasping this concept has been an integral part of my own journey toward accepting myself unconditionally. When I left my marketing job in 2000, it was with the understanding that I needed to take some time to learn how to be the person I was rather than just jumping into another situation that would make me feel important and needed. As you might imagine, this was a very challenging process—I'd be lying if I said it was easy. But with each new day, I began to recognize that I had the right to be more than just a "marketing" person or a "thin" person or any other type of person. I realized for the first time that I had a right to just be...me.

The more I could accept *being* who I was, the more I found myself interested in exploring things I truly enjoyed. For so long I had limited my choices to what everyone else thought was important. Now I was able to freely choose what made me feel happy and at peace.

While I'm not suggesting that we should all drop responsibility on its head so that we can seek out our inner person, it is sometimes helpful to take a step back from the busy-ness of life and explore how much of our day is spent doing instead of being. Learning to "be" frees us to make choices based on what is best for the growth and enrichment of ourselves and those around us, and it brings us one step closer to the balance we need.

Finding Balance

Recently I was told by a very smart businessman that people don't want balance. "Sure they do," I argued, to which he replied, "Not really—most people just want it all." And when I considered our human nature, I had to admit that Jim was right. But that doesn't mean that balance is not something to be desired. We just need to be reminded of the beautiful role it can play in our lives.

Balance is all around us. In the creative world, the gifted artist achieves a perfect balance of color and expression, leaving just enough room for the imagination of the viewer to add the final touch. A skilled musician combines melody, harmony, and lyric in a delicate balance that creates the platform for an emotional experience, and the most sought-after interior designers employ balance to give a room the feeling of beauty and comfort while creating a functional living space. Just as balance is necessary for all of these things, it is also the key to allowing us to live life more fully.

To find balance in our own lives, we must first take the extremes we live by and counter them with truth. For example, weighing our desire to be thin against the joy of having a well-nourished body. Or feeling good about our appearance, but not depending upon it as our measure of self-worth. Balance means taking the truth, both negative and positive, and finding a place where both aspects can exist in unity.

I believe in the life-changing power of *finding balance* so much that I've used that term as the foundation for everything I'm now doing. In seeking balance, we give ourselves new criteria for life that is often more forgiving and definitely more rewarding than the messages and demands of our culture.

So What?

By understanding that who we are is more important than what we do, we can find the balance that will help us walk toward freedom.

Action Steps

1. Take a moment to consider whether you are "willing to be willing" to change your thoughts about eating and weight. When you are ready, pray this simple prayer:

    God, I don't know that I'm ready to change yet,
    but I am willing to be willing.
    Please help me take the next step toward finding a place of balance
    with my approach to eating and weight control.
    I want to be free.

2. In the left-hand column below, write down the "Extremes" you live by, such as "Don't eat fat" or "Exercise every day." When you have written down as many as you can think of, use the right-hand column to counter each extreme with "Truth," such as "My body needs fat to operate well" or "A day of rest each week would be good for my soul."

    Extremes   *Truth*

Chapter 25

Changing Our Perspective

The real voyage of discovery consists not in seeking new landscapes, but
in having new eyes.

—MARCEL PROUST

As we discussed in chapter 20, we can find incredible freedom when we realize that so much of how we see ourselves depends upon our perspective.
With this truth in mind, an important next step is to begin the process of adjusting and broadening our narrow ideas about weight and food.

Adjusting Our Perception of Thin

As we discussed earlier, when we begin to consider breaking out of our cage, it is
natural to fear that doing so will require us to accept getting "fat." While it is
unlikely that we are going to become obese simply by coming off our weird diets,
we need to begin adjusting our perception of thin so that we will leave room for
ourselves to gain a few pounds for the sake of good health and balanced eating.

This was an important step for me in my own recovery. At the peak of my
disorder, I considered anything over a size 2 "fat." To prepare myself for the possibility of gaining weight, I began to look objectively at other women to get a
more accurate idea of what a normal body looked like. As I studied the land-
scape, I noticed a lot of women who carried quite a bit more weight than I did.
But in spite of the fact that they were a few sizes larger than I was, many of the
women I saw would be considered quite attractive by most people. These observations became my armor as I put on a little weight. As I grew out of a size 2,

and then out of a 4, I reminded myself that as long as my body was healthy and I felt good, the size I wore didn't really matter.

I knew I had truly made progress the day I bought something in a size 7/8. I had taken a 5/6 into the dressing room, but when it didn't fit, I calmly and confidently asked the salesperson for the next size up. As I waited for her to return, I considered that just a couple years earlier, I would have been horrified to say 7/8 aloud, yet suddenly I had no problem with the number. It was then that I realized I had successfully adjusted my perception of thin, enlarging it to accept a wider range of sizes and weight. Interestingly, being able to ask calmly for a *larger* size made me feel more in control than when I used to have to ask for a *smaller* size. It was strange, but the ability to accept whatever size fit best and be content with it made me realize that I was actually in a better place than the women who were always obsessed with getting thinner.

I realize that for many women a 7/8 seems quite small and that my struggle to accept this size could come across as ridiculous and even offensive. But all of us have different ideals when it comes to our weight and size. The important thing is to come to a point where we can adjust our ideal to allow ourselves to accept our bodies as they naturally are: fat, thin, or in-between.

As I've continued to walk this out, I have learned that it is *how* we wear our clothes—the confidence with which we carry ourselves—that says so much more about who we are than the actual number on the tag. This concept has freed me from the bondage of thinking that each time I go shopping I must be a size smaller. Now trips to the mall can include a gyro sandwich or a slice of pizza, guilt-free!

And having been on the other side of the fence for so long, I can definitely say the grass is greener on the side that's being fed.

Reevaluating the Way We Eat

Just as our perception of thin has been skewed, so has our idea of what it means to eat right. As we move toward allowing ourselves the "luxury" of a balanced diet, we need to reevaluate the role of food in our lives.

Rule No. 1: Throw Out the Rules!

Let's face it: Most of us have gotten pretty good at establishing rules about what we eat. We know the pros and especially the cons of all the foods that are out there, and after years of adhering to our own strict rules about off-limits, safe, and even reward foods, we can find it difficult to figure out what it even means to eat normally.

When it comes to learning how to eat again, we must first throw out all of our self-imposed rules and allow ourselves to consider new information about how our body handles food.

For example, I spent many years drastically limiting my fat intake because I believed that eating any kind of fat would make me gain weight. Because of this, it took me awhile to adjust to the idea that if I ate a cheeseburger, I wasn't going to gain several pounds overnight. As I cautiously began allowing myself the occasional burger or slice of pizza, I was surprised to see that my weight didn't suddenly balloon out of control. I also noticed that I started feeling more satisfied with my meals and less paranoid about eating and weight. I once thought that eating fat made me fat. Now I know that unless I overeat, my body is going to metabolize and use the fat I eat to make me stronger and healthier.

The truth is, we can—and should—allow ourselves to eat all types of foods. Many of us did so as children, and our bodies usually responded appropriately. That said, we need to look at what it means to eat wisely. For instance, we may want to consider the size of our portions or be careful about eating certain foods—like sugar—that might trigger unhealthy eating patterns. Taking our time as we learn to eat again will help us successfully begin incorporating normal foods back into our diet.

How Much Should I Eat?

For disordered eaters, the advice "Eat when you're hungry and stop when you're full" is problematic for a number of reasons. First of all, many of us are terrified of eating to the point of feeling full. We believe that doing so is a sign of failure, and our fear can often trigger us into a binge, a diet, or other unhealthy behaviors. So until we are ready to be more comfortable with feeling full, the advice to eat until we're full can actually cause a setback in our recovery.

Second, those who chronically diet require only a small amount of food to feel full. I often experienced this when I was first trying to eat better. I would genuinely feel full after only eating a few bites of food. Had I followed the advice to "stop when you're full," I would have continued eating less than my body needed and would never have been able to increase my food intake to a more healthy point.

A third problem with this advice is that many who binge, purge, or yo-yo diet have a hard time distinguishing between feeling hungry or full. For these individuals, portions might be too large or too small, and they won't even realize it.

When it comes to relearning portion sizes, I have found it helpful to look around at how much other people of average weight are eating. While I recognize that people's individual appetites can be quite different, considering the eating habits of several people makes it easier to gauge what a normal portion might be.

By beginning to incorporate normal portions back into our eating habits, we can slowly retrain our body to more easily recognize the feelings of hunger and satiety. Once this happens, it becomes easier to depend on our feelings of hunger and fullness as a gauge for how much we should eat.

When Should I Eat?

When it comes to determining *when* and *how often* we should eat, I think it's important to find a balance between the rigidity of a *schedule* and the freedom of a *routine.* These words are very similar, but to me they mean two different things.

A scheduled eater says, "I must eat only at 7:00, 12:00, and 5:00, and if I'm late for one of these times, then I must skip eating." For this person, every moment of the day is planned around mealtimes.

On the other hand, the goal of a routine eater is to eat meals at regular intervals, without crossing over into an obsession about specific times of the day eating is "allowed." For example, my routine is to eat breakfast when I first get up (whatever time that is), eat lunch sometime around the middle of the day, and then have dinner with my husband when he gets home from work. I don't worry about specific times other than to make sure I don't skip a meal altogether. If I am hungry between meals, I'll have a snack. If it's getting close to dinnertime, I'll try not to snack because I know that if I do I might be too full to eat the nutritious meal my body needs.

If dinner plans involve meeting friends later in the evening, I don't get all worked up about whether I'm going to gain weight by eating so late. Because I'm not stressed about the time of our meal, I am less likely to allow my food choices to be dictated by my fears and am less prone to eating more (or less) than I need to. This approach is less specific about when I can and can't eat and is focused more on making sure I eat regularly.

When it comes to how often we should eat, there are different schools of thought. For some people, eating three meals a day works well. They can easily plan meals around work or other demands, and by resisting the urge to snack in between, they increase their stomach's natural ability to feel hungry when it is mealtime. This is particularly helpful for those who are trying to get their appetite back into good working order.

Others prefer eating several small meals throughout the day. This prevents blood-sugar levels from plummeting between meals, which helps people feel less hungry and edgy and less likely to overeat (or undereat) at their next meal.

When considering how to plan your meals, try both of these methods and see what works best for you. I have seen the benefits of both—it just comes down to what fits your lifestyle and your physical needs best.

Food Logs—Pros and Cons

Food logs can be a helpful way to determine whether we are getting the nutrition we need. The tricky thing about them is that they can also trigger continued obsession. Early in my recovery a friend recommended that I use a food log to get a better idea of how much I was eating. As I began recording the calories, fat grams, and protein in everything I ate, I was surprised to discover that I still wasn't eating enough. While this was certainly helpful information, the detailed process of listing my meals made me fixate even more on my diet, which was exactly what I was trying to break free from. When I would see my total caloric intake climb for a few days, I found myself going back into restrictive mode again to make up for it. I ended up discontinuing the log until I got pregnant and had a more urgent need to make sure my body was getting what it needed. This time, however, instead of keeping track of calories and fat grams, I focused on tracking which food groups I was eating. I found this approach to be much more helpful and less likely to trigger obsessive thinking.

Even with this more positive experience behind me, I still prefer not to use a log. I can certainly see the advantages of using such a tool—for the right type of person. As with using a scale, the important thing is to determine whether a log is going to be a help or a hindrance. We have to honestly ask ourselves, "What am I going to do with the information?"

Vitamins and Supplements

Since disordered eating often robs our body of the nutrients found naturally in food, it is wise to consider taking some vitamin supplements as part of our new balanced diet. I'm certainly no expert on these, but it is commonly believed that formulas containing natural ingredients seem to be absorbed best by the body. If you are unsure as to what supplements you might need, check with a nutritionist or dietitian. Be sure to tell this person how you've been eating so that he or she can have the best possible shot at determining what your body might be missing in the way of nutrients and vitamins.

So What?

Much of our toiling comes from the fact that our perception of what is thin—and thus acceptable—is incredibly narrow. Allowing ourselves to broaden our perspective about who we are and what we can eat gives us the freedom to make choices based on a larger range of options.

Action Steps

1. Take a trip to a public place and spend some time looking at all the different body types. When you see a woman you think looks attractive and healthy, honestly consider the size of her body as compared to yours. If you have a difficult time accurately judging size, bring a friend or your husband with you. Now consider how much more fun it would be to be able to eat normally if only you were willing to allow yourself a wider range of what is an acceptable weight. Write your thoughts here.

2. If possible, make an appointment to see a nutritionist who can get you started on a healthy eating plan. Make sure it's someone with whom you're comfortable and whose approach is balanced. Set a target date for your visit and write it here:

3. Try slowly incorporating into your diet foods that used to be off-limits. Be mindful of certain foods that you know could trigger a binge, but give yourself permission to eat something you like. Gradually, you will discover that eating is enjoyable again. As your body gets back into the groove of metabolizing a wider variety of foods, you will find that you feel healthier and are more able to enjoy life.

"Some foods I would like to give myself permission to eat are":

Opening the Closet Door

We are only as weak as our biggest secret.

—a recovering alcoholic in Tennessee

O ne of the most pivotal moments in my journey toward freedom was when I finally found the courage to crack open the door of my closet, letting in just enough light to begin seeing the truth behind the lies I had believed for so long. At first it seemed a terribly scary proposition to admit my own weakness to someone else, but I quickly came to see the benefits of my decision.

Finding a Confidant

As a proudly independent child, I used to look with disdain upon other kids I knew who would seek out the school counselor for guidance on particular issues. *I don't need anyone else's advice,* I haughtily thought to myself. *Besides, what can they tell me that I don't already know?*

It was this same foolish pride that for many years fueled my belief that it would be wrong or weak to seek out a professional counselor to talk with about my eating. Part of my apprehension was founded in truth—it seemed that there weren't very many who understood where I was coming from—but it was also the stigma I had attached to the whole idea of therapy that kept me from seeking out help sooner than I did.

When I first met Susi, it was after a few years of coming to terms not only with my eating but also with some other issues in my life. Even though it still seemed terribly self-indulgent to spend an entire hour talking about myself to someone I hardly knew, I began to understand that it was okay for me to do so. One day I told Susi that it was hard for me not to feel selfish when spewing out all my problems to her, and she gently reminded me that this process was not only acceptable but necessary to my recovery. And she was right. Looking back, I can see that if it hadn't been for Susi and our weekly sessions, I would never be where I am today.

Not Just Anyone Will Do

When it comes to seeking out a listening ear and balanced advice, I can't stress enough the importance of finding someone who will address the *real* issue instead of getting bogged down in the details of food logs and weight charts. While these tools certainly have their place, it was the opportunity to get at the root, not the symptoms, of my problem that was so life changing for me.

A lot of well-intentioned people wish to give advice but don't have what it takes to draw us out in a way that shines light on the root of our problem. Because of this, it is important to know that you have the right to discontinue seeing someone if you feel it's just not helping you. Too often I hear from women who are trapped in dead-end therapy because they feel too guilty to end the relationship. But no one benefits in such a situation. In this case, it is better to make a mistake, admit it, and get out than to feel compelled to remain in what might not be a healthy or productive therapy environment. When you're looking for the right person to talk to, it's important to have some criteria in mind.

Things to look for:
- Can you trust this therapist completely?
- Do you feel this therapist is genuinely interested in helping you?
- Does this therapist speak your "language" or is he or she always talking over your head?
- If spirituality is important to you, does this therapist incorporate that into his or her approach?
- Do you feel you can be completely honest with this therapist?
- Does this therapist challenge you to seek truth?

- Does he or she challenge you to think through the issues?
- Does he or she have some experience with disordered eaters?
- Does he or she have an understanding of the important role nutrition must play in your recovery?

Things to be cautious of:
- *A therapist who is too eager to prescribe medication.* Sometimes therapists prescribe medication before spending adequate time with us to fully understand our issues. While certain medications have helped with some eating disorders, it is also important to look at root issues and the overall person.
- *Treatment that is too focused on one aspect of the problem.* Successfully treating disordered eating and other unhealthy behaviors involves placing equal focus on the emotional, spiritual, physical, and mental aspects of our issues. Too much emphasis placed on any one dimension can do more harm than good. The key is balance.
- *A tendency to be too eager to assign blame.* Again, the key here is balance. I learned through my discussions with Susi that events in my past had contributed to my disordered behavior, but to simply blame these things would have robbed me of the opportunity to accept responsibility for the choices I have made and continue to make.

These are just a few suggestions. Trust your heart to guide you in making the decision about who is best able to give you the help you need.

Therapist, Counselor, or Friend?

While the role of a friend or spouse is indispensable when we're walking through any life challenge, I think that in most cases a trained therapist or counselor is going to be best equipped to give sound advice while maintaining healthy professional boundaries. The trick here is to understand that just because someone has a degree hanging on the wall doesn't mean that he or she is going to be the right person to help you. This is why it's important to go into any such relationship with an I'm-going-to-try-this-out-and-see-if-it-feels-right approach. I would suggest that you address this plan on the first visit so that you give your-self the option to move on if, after a fair evaluation, you feel the therapy is not working for you.

That said, it's important to know the difference between bad therapy and therapy that makes you feel bad. These are two very different things. If your ses-sions make you feel uncomfortable, that doesn't necessarily mean they're not helping. This discomfort could be just what you need to get at the ugly roots of your problem. Consider this distinction carefully before making a change, since several sessions are often needed to be able to determine whether therapy is working.

If it is not feasible for you to seek out a professional counselor, consider care-fully whether a trusted friend might be willing to be a voice of reason for you as you take this journey toward healing. In his book *Hope, Help, and Healing for Eating Disorders,* Dr. Gregory Jantz offers some good suggestions for what to look for in such a person:

"Helper" Criteria
  1. They must realize it is not their job to "fix" you.
  2. They should operate from a position of acceptance, not condemna-tion or judgment.
  3. They should try to read up on the subject of eating disorders, espe-cially the EDNOS category.
  4. They should not try to minimize your pain.
  5. They should be willing to just listen and provide comfort instead of thinking they must always have an answer.
  6. They should try to accept your version of past events even if they remember them differently. They should also give you time and permission to be angry.
  7. They should not try to be your "warden," policing your actions or making demands.
  8. They should be willing to honestly share their opinions but allow room for you to have a differing view.

9. They must understand that you need time to work through this
    properly.[1]

I know that this is a rather long list and that no helper is perfect, but once
you find someone you think might be able to fill this role in your life, go over
this list with them so that he or she can know where you're coming from.

In my own experience, I asked God to bring someone into my life to help
me, and a few weeks later I met Susi. So if you've already tried finding help on
your own and were unsuccessful, or if you aren't sure just where to turn, ask God
to provide someone you can talk to.

Going Public

One day I was pouring myself a cup of coffee in preparation for another long
meeting at the company where I worked. I had been out sick for a few days, and
while I was in the kitchen I bumped into the president of our company who
asked me how I was feeling. I told him I was getting better, and he asked whether
I might have a chronic illness of some sort, since I seemed to be under the
weather quite often. Looking back on our conversation, I still can't fathom
where these next words came from.

"No," I said. "The truth is, I just don't eat enough."

Now I'd done it.

He looked at me quizzically, "Oh, uh, do you just not like to eat…or…?"

"Well," I replied, "I guess I'm just afraid to eat, because I don't want to get
fat."

I think my comment took us both by surprise.

Suddenly I was buzzing inside, partially from the fear that my value in the
company was going to plummet now that I had admitted to being imperfect,
but mostly from the euphoria of speaking the truth after years of lying to myself
and everyone around me.

This was a *big* moment for me. A definite "coming out"—facing my fear of
rejection and realizing that it was time to be honest, for *me*. After all, this was
finally about me, not anyone else. It was about being able to look at myself

without the rose-colored glasses and see that I was worthy of love in spite of my flaws.

The best part is that my monumental confession didn't seem to faze anyone. They didn't gather behind closed doors and scheme plans for my removal. They didn't whisper to each other, "Did you hear about Constance? She's really got a problem. She must not be that good at marketing after all. I mean, did you hear that she's afraid to get fat???"

In fact, very few people could really appreciate the personal hell I was living in, as I saw in the way they casually brushed aside my "big" news so they could get on to more pressing matters. Suddenly I felt free as a bird. With the weight of my secret lifted from my chest, I finally had room to breathe.

A few months later when I turned in my resignation, Peter thanked me for being so open with him that day in the kitchen. Since then I've come to realize that a willingness to tell the truth, even when it's not pretty, is a helpful thing for others who are on their own journey of self-discovery.

After all, each one of us has things we struggle to break free from—for me it was an eating disorder, for others it might be alcohol addiction or pornography or an unhealthy focus on accomplishments. Whatever our struggle, by choosing to be honest, we become light in a dark place, and as we are light to others, we light our own world, too.

A Word of Caution

Before you rush out and proclaim your secret to the world, bear in mind a couple of things. First, it is important to wait until you're sure you feel ready to live outside the lie. Not everyone is going to know what to do with the information you share with them—some may think it's their job to hold you accountable for how you feel about your weight. Others may feel responsible to make sure you eat enough or don't eat too much. The good news is that for the most part, people are going to love and support you and not pay a whole lot more attention to your problem than they used to, but it's important to be prepared for those who aren't so enlightened.

Who Needs to Know?

For many of us, our family is a good place to start. Even with its flaws, the family environment is probably a safe place to start being honest. You alone, however, can determine whether your family will be able to respond to your news in a positive way. If there are members of your family who could be a trigger for you, then don't involve them in the process until you know you're ready.

After telling family members, a logical sequence would be to include close friends and eventually, if you so desire, those you spend most of your time with: your coworkers.

But don't feel that it's your duty to become accountable to these people. The point is to begin learning how to accept yourself without depending upon the approval of others.

So What?

There is no shame in admitting we don't have it all together. By finding someone who can help us deal with our issues and walk toward being honest with those we are close to, we remove from the equation the fear of their disapproval and allow for the possibility that they might actually accept us just as we are.

Action Steps

1. Take a moment to consider who might be someone you could seek counsel from regarding your eating and weight issues. Write some ideas down here.

2. Set a goal for when you plan to make an appointment to talk with this
    person (i.e., this week, this month). Write the date here.

3. When considering going public about your eating disorder, you need to
    evaluate who may or may not be the right people to tell. Make a list of a
    few people you feel you can trust with your secret. When you are ready,
    make a plan to be honest with them.

Anticipating the Pitfalls

Let him who desires peace prepare for war.

—VEGETIUS (fourth century A.D.)

It's been several years now since I first prayed my willing-to-be-willing prayer. In that time I've sought—and found—good counsel. I've attended support groups. I've explored my past and questioned my future. I've become a mother and faced my fear of gaining weight and losing thinness. I've wrestled with the elements of my human nature that drive me in my quest for the approval of others. I've learned that how I look is not as important as the big picture of why I'm here on this earth. Yet even with all of this progress, I remain acutely aware of the need to anticipate the pitfalls of my own recovery process.

Counteracting Our Triggers

To effectively guard against falling back into unhealthy patterns, we must be aware of what triggers those patterns and make plans for counteracting the triggers when they come up. In chapter 16 you listed many of your own triggers. Keep this list somewhere close so that you can refer back to it often. When you find yourself feeling worthless because of external factors or toying with the idea of restricting your diet a little, look at your list and see if any of your trigger points have been touched on recently.

For example, one of my triggers used to be fashion magazines. If I came across a copy of *Vogue* or *W,* I would find myself immediately unhappy with my body. For a while my strategy to counteract this trigger was to avoid these kinds of magazines entirely. Removing this trigger gave me time to continue developing a stronger sense of self-acceptance. As I got further along in my recovery, I eventually reached a point where this trigger was no longer a problem for me. I still find myself drawn to fashion magazines, but I have no problem looking objectively now at the images of beauty they portray. I know I don't have to look like the models.

As you progress in your own journey, actively look for ways to counteract your triggers. If you are triggered by stress, find an activity that provides a good outlet for you. If you are triggered by sugar or certain foods, be careful how you approach incorporating them into your diet. For each and every trigger you've listed, try listing a method to counteract it. (This exercise appears at the end of this chapter.)

Arming Ourselves with Truth

Sometimes removing a trigger from our lives is not an option. For instance, we may not be able to separate ourselves from our job environment or our social setting. In these situations, our best option for countering the trigger is to arm ourselves with truth. Following are some truths that have made the biggest difference in my life:

• Choosing to gain or maintain is just as valid as choosing to lose.
• Sex appeal does not equal true acceptance.
• God cares more about who I am than what I weigh.
• That which defines me controls me.
• Everyone has a different definition of fat, thin, attractive, and perfect.
• Living to inspire is more fulfilling than living to impress.
• True reality is often different than I think it is.
• A richer life awaits me outside the cage.

In moments of weakness, there is no shame in needing a reminder of these and other truths. You may want to go back through this book and highlight the truths that speak the most to you. (At the end of this chapter there is room for you to list these as well.)

Finding a Voice of Reason

Even with knowing these and other truths, we must be prepared for moments of fear and insecurity that will try to lure us back into the false comfort of our cages. During such times, it is important to have someone in mind who can be our voice of reason.

For me this has often been my husband. It is not unusual for me to check in with him from time to time to get an honest view of how I'm doing. Since he is able to look at me more objectively than I can, he's a safe person to turn to when I'm convinced my butt has grown larger overnight.

Just the other day I saw a woman who was several sizes larger than I, and I asked my husband, "How would you feel if I was that size?" to which he replied, "Um, the same, I think…" These little check-ins are good for me. The healthier I get in my thinking, the less I need them, but they're still an important part of my continued recovery.

One Day at a Time

So many people have used this phrase that it's become cliché in our culture, but there is an important and timeless principle here. As with any other journey, we have only to take this one day at a time. We don't need to make up for yesterday with today. And if we fail today, we still have tomorrow and the next day and the next day after that.

What is important is not our success or failure on any particular day but our decision to keep moving forward and to keep seeking victory. No matter our circumstances, we never have to be further from freedom than where we stand today. Now that we know the truth, we can choose to move forward.

So What?

By being aware of potential pitfalls and arming ourselves with truth, we can be victorious in the fight for self-acceptance. This victory allows us to live more fully, delighting in the freedom to eat, to accept our body's natural size, and most of all, to enjoy life outside the cage.

Action Steps

1. In chapter 16, you made a list of your triggers—review it now and write down some of the most difficult ones in the left-hand column. In the right-hand column, write down some strategies to counteract the triggers.

    My Most Difficult Triggers   *Strategies to Counteract Them*

2. Many truths have been presented in this book. Think about the one(s) that have had the most impact on you, and write them below. Refer back to this page when you need a reminder of the truths that can set you free.

    Truth 1: _____

    Truth 2: _____

Truth 3: _____

Truth 4: _____

Truth 5: _____

Truth 6: _____

Truth 7: _____

Truth 8: _____

Truth 9: _____

Truth 10: _____

Prayer

*God, thank you for helping me
be willing to get this far.*

*Please be with me each day as I consciously remind myself
to accept myself the way you made me.*

*I know in my heart that freedom is something I desire;
help me hold to this truth as I walk forward out of the cage.*

Thank you.

Final Thoughts

Even though I have made a lot of progress, I would be lying if I said that I no longer struggle. I do not say this to steal your hope, for I am incredibly hopeful for continued change. But it's important to know that leaving a life of disordered eating and weight obsession is a process, not a quick fix.

There are exciting times—moments when things become black and white, and a little spot of truth suddenly brings great clarity to our vision. And then there are discouraging times when we fall back into frustrating patterns. Each step, positive and negative, is necessary in creating a balanced foundation for deliberate and sustainable change.

I can tell you from personal experience that life outside the cage is much more worth living. Joys await you that you won't experience until you decide to break free from the lies that have held you in fear. Throughout this book we've discussed the many ways our lives would be different if not for our obsession. Look at your own list and consider whether you desire those things enough to take some bold steps.

I can also tell you that my faith has been very important to me through this process. It is my belief that God wants what's best for me that has helped me trust him and choose to walk toward freedom. For me, there is something universally significant that occurs when you realize you need not walk alone. But in the end, you must learn these truths for yourself, for it is only in knowing them personally that you can apply them to your life.

It is my prayer that reading this book has brought you one step closer to seeking such truth and to finding the courage to reclaim your right to your body and your life.

Notes

Chapter 2: When Dieting Turns Chronic

1. Leanne Spencer, e-mail correspondence, May 2002.

2. Spencer, e-mail correspondence, May 2002.

3. From www.anred.com/stats.html.

4. Christopher G. Fairburn and G. Terence Wilson, *Binge Eating: Nature, Assessment and Treatment* (New York: Guildford Press, 1993), 11.

5. Sharon Hersh, personal interview, March 2002.

6. Leanne Spencer, personal interview, April 2002.

7. Dr. Alan Schwitzer, personal interview, April 2002.

8. Katherine A. Beals, "Subclinical Eating Disorders in Female Athletes," *Journal of Physical Education, Recreation and Dance* 71, no. 7 (September 2000): 23.

9. C. M. Shisslak, M. Crago, and L. S. Estes, "The Spectrum of Eating Disturbances," *International Journal of Eating Disorders* 18, no. 3 (November 1995): 209.

10. J. H. Linner, "Comparative Effectiveness of Gastric Bypass and Gastroplasty: A Clinical Study," *Archives of Surgery* 117 (1982): 695-700, quoted in J. F. Wilber, "Obesity: The Role of Gastric Surgery" (Letter to the Editor), *Journal of the American Medical Association* 266, no. 22 (11 December 1991): 3130.

11. F. D. Kurtzman et al., "Eating Disorders Among Selected Female Populations at UCLA," *Journal American Dietetic Association* 89, no. 1 (January 1989): 45.

12. S. Rubinstein and B. Caballero, "Is Miss America an Undernourished Role Model?" *Journal of the American Medical Association* 283, no. 12 (22 March 2000): 1569.

13. From www.healthywithin.com/stats.htm.

14. From www.healthywithin.com/stats.htm.

15. Toni Luppino, "Yo-Yo Dieting: Early Education Is the Key in the Potentially Fatal Gain-Lose Weight Cycle," *American Fitness* 10, no. 4 (July/August 1992): 60-1.

16. Luppino, "Yo-Yo Dieting," 60-1.

17. J. D. Heyman, "Hollywood's Obsession with Weight," *US Weekly* (19 March 2001): 52.

18. Leanne Spencer, e-mail correspondence, May 2002.

19. Dr. Harry Gwirtsman, personal interview, July 2002.

20. To read this report, see Sharlene Hesse-Biber, "Report on a Panel Longitudinal Study of College Women's Eating Patterns and Eating Disorders: Noncontinuum Versus Continuum Measures," *Healthy Care for Women International* 13 (1992): 375-91.

21. Sharlene Hesse-Biber, personal interview, September 2002.

22. Sharlene Hesse-Biber, personal interview, September 2002.

23. R. L. Pyle et al., "Maintenance, Treatment and Six Month Outcome for Bulimic Patients Who Respond to Initial Treatment," *American Journal of Psychiatry* 147 (1990): 871-5.

Chapter 3: The Thought Process

1. Sharon Hersh, personal interview, March 2002.

Chapter 4: Weird Eating—Exposed

1. Dorie Edelstein, "Dangerous Dieting," *Ladies' Home Journal* (June 2002): 72.

2. From www.anred.com/defslesser.html.

3. *Rock Bodies,* VH1 and *Self* magazine, 2 September 2002 broadcast.

4. *Rock Bodies,* 2 September 2002.

Chapter 6: We Live in a Fallen World

1. Leanne Spencer, e-mail correspondence, June 2002.

2. Sharlene Hesse-Biber, *Am I Thin Enough Yet? The Cult of Thinness and the Commercialization of Identity* (New York: Oxford University Press, 1996), 9.

3. Those who follow the Atkins Diet constantly check their urine to ensure they are in a state of ketosis, "a condition in which the body will turn to fat for fuel and is producing ketones as a by-product." The diet advocates remaining in a state of constant ketosis for ultimate results.

Chapter 7: How Our Past Shaped Us

1. L. Mellin, C. E. Irwin Jr., and S. Scully, "Prevalence of Disordered Eating in Girls: A Survey of Middle Class Children," *Journal of the American Dietetic Association* 92, no. 7 (July 1992): 851.

2. From www.healthywithin.com/stats.htm.

3. Sharlene Hesse-Biber, *Am I Thin Enough Yet? The Cult of Thinness and the Commercialization of Identity* (New York: Oxford University Press, 1996), 101.

4. Dr. Phillip C. McGraw, "Kids and Weight" NBC, 18 September 2002 broadcast.

Chapter 8: Significant Life Events

1. Dr. Donald R. Durham, personal interview, April 2002.

2. Mary Pipher, Ph.D., *Reviving Ophelia: Saving the Selves of Adolescent Girls* (New York: Ballantine, 1994), 170.

3. Michelle Stacey, "Fear of Pregnancy: Is It the Way Our Bodies Change—or How Our Lives Will Change—That Sometimes Scares Us?" (Body Language), *Shape* 21, no. 9 (May 2002): 94.

4. Jane Greer, Ph.D., *Gridlock: Finding the Courage to Move On in Love, Work and Life* (New York: Doubleday, 2000), quoted in *Ladies' Home Journal* (June 2002): 63.

Chapter 9: My Body Has Betrayed Me

1. Nicole Johnson, e-mail correspondence, September 2002.

2. From www.anred.com/diab.html.

3. Sharlene Hesse-Biber, *Am I Thin Enough Yet? The Cult of Thinness and the Commercialization of Identity* (New York: Oxford University Press, 1996), 82.

4. Julia Ross, *The Diet Cure* (New York: Viking, 1999), 200.

Chapter 10: Challenging Environments

1. Dominique Andrews, "Better Neighborhood, Worse Body Image," *Ladies' Home Journal* (June 2002): 70.

2. Katherine A. Beals, "Subclinical Eating Disorders in Female Athletes," *Journal of Physical Education, Recreation and Dance* 71, no. 7 (September 2000): 23.

3. Beals, "Subclinical Eating Disorders," 23.

4. Nora Underwood, "Body Envy: Thin Is In, and People Are Messing with Mother Nature As Never Before," *Macleans* (14 August 2000): 36.

5. John Monahan, "Supermodel Carre Otis Finds the Greatest Gift of All," *Better Nutrition* (May 2002), 36-8.

6. Emily Sohn, "The Hunger Artists: Are Genes and Brain Chemistry at the Root of Eating Disorders?" *U.S. News & World Report* (10 June 2002): 45-50.

Chapter 11: The Hollywood Effect

1. J. D. Heyman, "Hollywood's Obsession with Weight," *US Weekly* (19 March 2001): 54.

2. Heyman, "Hollywood's Obsession," 52.

3. Michelle Tauber et al., "Learning Curves," *Sunday Express* (2000), quoted in *People* (4 April 2002): 95-6.

4. W. Keck, "*Ally McBeal's* Courtney Thorne-Smith Says She's Fed Up with the Pressure to Be Thin," *US Weekly,* no. 304 (11 December 2000), 32.

5. Amy Wallace, "True Thighs," *MORE* (September 2002): 90-4.

6. Tauber, "Learning Curves," 96.

7. Tauber, "Learning Curves," 101.

8. Tauber, "Learning Curves," 98.

9. Marisa Cohen, "Real Women Have Curves," *Glamour* (July 2002): 129.

10. Cohen, "Real Women Have Curves," 129.

Chapter 13: Making Choices out of Fear

1. Andrea Morris, "Permission to Eat," *Elle* 17, no. 11 (July 2001): 84.

2. Morris, "Permission to Eat," 84.

3. Jill Malden, quoted in Morris, "Permission to Eat," 84.

4. Dr. Donald R. Durham, personal interview, April 2002.

Chapter 14: We're Addicted

1. Debbie Danowski and Pedro Lazaro, M.D., *Why Can't I Stop Eating?* (Center City, Minn.: Hazelden, 2000), 5.

2. Danowski and Lazaro, *Why Can't I Stop Eating?* 5.

3. Julia Ross, *The Diet Cure* (New York: Viking, 1999), 33.

4. Ross, *The Diet Cure,* 33.

5. Sharlene Hesse-Biber, *Am I Thin Enough Yet? The Cult of Thinness and the Commercialization of Identity* (New York: Oxford University Press, 1996), 67.

Chapter 16: Triggers

1. From www.healthywithin.com/stats.htm.

2. Tracy White, personal interview, May 2002.

3. Alanis Morissette, "That I Would Be Good," from the album *Supposed Former Infatuation Junkie,* Maverick Records, 1998.

4. India.Arie, "Video," from the album *Acoustic Soul,* Motown Records, 2001.

5. Pink, "Don't Let Me Get Me," from the album *Missundaztood,* Arista, 2001.

6. Robert Lefever, M.D., and Marie Shafe, "Brain Chemistry: Combinations of Foods in the Blood Trigger Effects Very Similar to Alcohol," *Employee Assistance* 3, no. 8. (March 1991): n.p.

7. Dr. Donald R. Durham, personal interview, April 2002.

Chapter 18: Our Excuses and the Price We Pay

1. Dr. Gregory L. Jantz, personal interview, April 2002.

2. *Rock Bodies,* VH1 and *Self* magazine, 2 September 2002 broadcast.

3. J. X. Wang, "Body Mass and Probability of Pregnancy During Assisted Reproduction Treatment: Retrospective Study," *British Medical Journal* (25 November 2000).

4. Dr. C. Wayne Callaway, as referenced by Michelle Stacey, "Fear of Pregnancy: Is It the Way Our Bodies Change—Or How Our Lives Change—That Sometimes Scares Us?" (Body Language) *Shape* 21, no. 9 (May 2002): 94.

5. Silius Italicus (A.D. 26–101), Roman epic poet. *Punica,* 11:592-4.

6. Margo Maine, Ph.D., *Body Wars* (Carlsbad, Calif.: Gurze Books, 2000), 45.

7. Dr. Phillip C. McGraw, "Kids and Weight" NBC, 18 September 2002 broadcast.

Chapter 19: Sex Appeal Does Not Equal True Acceptance

1. Wendy Shalit, *A Return to Modesty* (New York: Touchstone, 1999), 170.

Chapter 21: On Getting Older

1. Sydney Smith, "Recipe for a Salad," *Lady Holland's Memoir* (1855), quoted in John M. Shanahan, ed., *The Most Brilliant Thoughts of All Time (In Two Lines or Less)* (New York: Cliff Street Books, 1999), 203.

Chapter 22: That Which Defines Us Controls Us

1. 1 Samuel 16:7.

Chapter 26: Opening the Closet Door

1. Material for "Helper Criteria" was adapted from Dr. Gregory L. Jantz, *Hope, Help, and Healing for Eating Disorders* (Colorado Springs: WaterBrook, 2002), 150-2.

About the Author

CONSTANCE RHODES is a former marketing director for Sparrow Records, a division of EMI. For more than a decade she struggled with disordered eating and chronic dieting. Today she is founder and director of FINDING*balance*, an organization designed to educate, inform, and inspire others in the areas of eating, image, and life management. She and her husband, AJ, live in Franklin, Tennessee, with their son, Christian.

If this book has inspired you to break free from a life of disordered eating, Constance would love to hear from you. You can write to her at:

FINDING*balance*
P.O. Box 284
Franklin, TN 37065
E-mail: breakingfree@findingbalance.com

Please visit her Web site at www.findingbalance.com for additional resources and information.

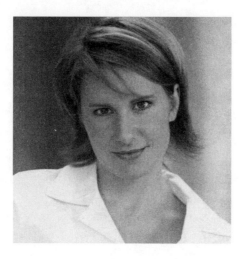

FINDINGbalance
eating image life

To learn more about Shaw Books and view our
catalog of products, log on to our Web site:
www.shawbooks.com

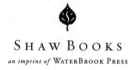

SHAW BOOKS
an imprint of WATERBROOK PRESS